Health Information
and Health Reform

Karen A. Duncan

Health Information and Health Reform

Understanding the Need for a National Health Information System

Jossey-Bass Publishers • San Francisco

Substantial discounts on bulk quantities of Jossey-Bass books are available to corporations, professional associations, and other organizations. For details and discount information, contact the special sales department at Jossey-Bass Inc., Publishers. (415) 433-1740; Fax (415) 433-0499.

For sales outside the United States, contact Maxwell Macmillan International Publishing Group, 866 Third Avenue, New York, New York 10022.

Manufactured in the United States of America. Nearly all Jossey-Bass books and jackets are printed on recycled paper containing at least 10 percent postconsumer waste, and many are printed with either soy- or vegetable-based ink, which emits fewer volatile organic compounds during the printing process than petroleum-based ink.

Library of Congress Cataloging-in-Publication Data

Duncan, K. A. (Karen A.)
    Health Information and health reform: understanding the need for
a national health information system / Karen A. Duncan. — 1st ed.
        p.   cm. — (The Jossey-Bass health series)
    Includes bibliographical references and index.
    ISBN 1-55542-659-X
    1. Medical informatics—United States. 2. Health care reform—
United States. I. Title. II. Series.
    R858.D86   1994
    610'.285—dc20   93-50693
                                                                      CIP

FIRST EDITION
HB Printing   10 9 8 7 6 5 4 3 2 1   *Code 9453*

The Jossey-Bass Health Series

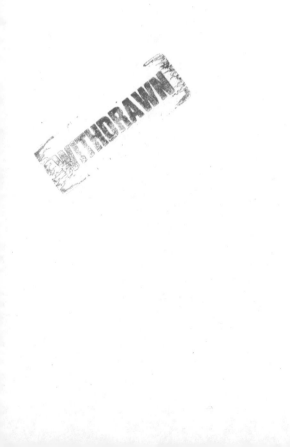

Contents

ix

Part Three:
Making Transformation a Reality

List of Figures

To my father,
Robert William Akins,
whose life experiences continue
to provide inspiration and insight

Preface

The U.S. health care system is in crisis, and the demand for reform is urgent. As is true of many other contemporary social systems, the workings of health care have become so complex that the resulting pervasive problems seem to defy understanding and solution. The contentiousness of today's reform debate underscores the need to look further for answers. True reform would encompass much more than changes in payment mechanisms and modes of delivery; it would be based on approaches that could reshape the evolutionary path of the system. To achieve reform, we need first to deepen our understanding of the complexity of the system and of the underlying forces that brought it into crisis.

Giving information technology—computers and communications technology—a key role in health care reform is an idea that will seem natural to health care professionals who have experienced the positive impact of the technology in institutions. However, the carefully planned and executed introduction of information technology on a national scale—as a National Health Information System—is a dramatic, expensive initiative that requires strong justification. The special point of view of this book is that, when we study the underlying forces that have shaped the health care system, the kinds of problems we find are those that are especially amenable to solution by means of information technology. Moreover, information technology is the ideal tool for redirecting those underlying forces so as to prevent future crises.

Health Information and Health Reform was written because health care professionals and decision makers have a particular need to understand the forces at work in the health care system and the potential of information as a basis for envisioning their roles in the system's evolution. The purpose of the book is to broaden that understanding, empowering leaders within the health care system to take the reform initiative. This is perhaps the first nontechnical book that explains why the system is in crisis and also the role of information technology in helping to alleviate the crisis and create the health care system of the future.

The book offers a framework for understanding the mission of the health care system and the forces that operate in and on the system. It further offers a second framework, a health care information framework, that provides the rationale for understanding how information technology is an enabling technology to transform the health care system in a most constructive way.

Audience for the Book

This book was written for people who are concerned about the future of the health care system. It is for health care professionals, administrators, and policy makers who know that their system does not work as well as it should and want to know why. They will find out how the system became what it is today and what will happen if we continue on our present path. They will learn how information technology can be a positive force for the health care system as a whole if its use is shaped by the health care professionals it is intended to serve.

Physician executives will learn about the emerging vital connection between clinical practice and health policy and about the important role they can play in shaping the future system. They will find justification for expanded use of information technology in clinical settings as an essential element of high-quality patient care.

Nurse executives will learn about the connection between the nursing care they manage today and the potential role of nursing in the information technology–based system of the future. The book shows that they can play a role in designing the national system and should strengthen their commitment to the computer-based patient record.

Health care administrators, who are already in the forefront of change, will find out what the next challenges on the health care reform horizon must be. They will see the need for their leadership in the evolution of the future health care system, as well as the need for cooperative rather than competitive development of the proposed National Health Information System.

Health care policy and decision makers will find out why the health care system must link up with the information age. They will come away with a better understanding of the forces behind the current crisis and how these forces are still operating to shape the future system. They will become better equipped to assess proposed reform approaches and ensure that reform is a win-win proposition for the health care system and the American people.

Health profession educators and students are an important audience for these ideas because they have the greatest opportunity and flexibility to make new ideas happen. I hope that this book will find its way into classrooms as a counterpoint to the status quo.

Medical informatics professionals who have questioned the relevance of their work to the health care system will find a special focus on their professional responsibility to work on real system problems. Here, they will learn just what those problems are.

For all these groups, the book uses a systems approach to make the vital connection between the problems of the health care system, the solutions, and the imperative to move the system into the information age.

Overview of Contents

Health Information and Health Reform first analyzes the crisis in health care and then advocates the use of information technology as a transforming agent. Since complex problems must be understood before they can be solved, Part One (Chapters One through Four) closely examines the evolution and nature of the current system.

Chapter One develops a picture of the range of crises in today's health care system, focusing particularly on the dissonance among stakeholders and the sheer complexity of the system.

Chapter Two discusses the values of society as the forces that should define the mission and set goals for the health care system. It then defines a mission and goals for health care that echo and guide analysis throughout the book. It also introduces some qualities of good systems according to general systems theory and assesses the health care system for these qualities, highlighting the inescapable interrelationships and interdependencies of the various stakeholders of the health care system.

Chapter Three draws a picture of the forces that have shaped the health care system over the past forty-odd years and that will continue to have a negative impact in the future unless the health care system intervenes on its own behalf. Chapter Four relates these forces to contemporary problems and shows why providers especially are powerless to change.

Part Two (Chapters Five through Eleven) explains how information flow holds the key to successful change and why information technology is an essential agent for change. Chapter Five shows how disruption in the flow of information of every kind—an *information logjam*—has prevented the health care system from keeping pace with the demands of modern society and from capitalizing on the benefits of its own technological successes.

Chapter Six explains how the health care system could function under *information liberation.* As a keystone to a future health care system, requirements for a conceptual *information framework for health care* are described in Chapter Seven. This chapter shows the critical nature of information flow among all elements of the system and beyond.

The essential information flow is incredibly complex, and it will be impossible to achieve without collaborative leadership in the health care system or without the extensive integration of computer and communications technology. Information technology concepts are introduced in a nontechnical way in Chapter Eight, and the way the technology has been used in health care is briefly discussed. Then the concepts of a National Health Information System are explained at increasing levels of complexity in Chapters Nine through Eleven, with special emphasis on the necessity for such a system and the safeguards it must contain. These chapters also show the relationship of institutional, local, and regional systems to the national system.

Part Three (Chapters Twelve through Fourteen) discusses progress toward a National Health Information System, the impact such a system could have in transforming health care, and how we could begin to achieve it. Chapter Twelve integrates the National Health Information System concepts and describes some ongoing work that could serve as building blocks. Chapter Thirteen shows how the future, transformed health care system might function after an environment of liberated information is established. The scenarios go far beyond showing what one can do with technology; they illustrate the transformation of the health care system that would be possible once information technology is fully integrated into health care.

Finally, Chapter Fourteen discusses the implications of trends in health care today and issues a wake-up call to potential leaders who can help put the course of health care reform on track.

Following the text, the Information Resources lists a number of associations, organizations, readings, and conferences that can give the interested reader a broader background on health policy and information technology in health care.

While this book is in some sense a gentle indictment of the health care system and especially of the physician establishment for its failure to lead, it is in no way an indictment of individual physicians and nurses who are doing their best to provide a complex and poorly understood service to those who need it.

Because the National Health Information System would cut across and support any legitimate reform process, a discussion of current proposals for reform is unwarranted. Too much has been written about *what* should be done and not enough about *why;* this book attempts to meet that need and give readers the tools with which they themselves can assess the more specific reform proposals.

Acknowledgments

I am especially grateful to my husband, George Glaser, for his loving support. I am also grateful to Nancy Karp, who supplied me with dozens of clippings and unflagging moral support; Roger Shannon, who shared seminal systems concepts; and Claire Pryor, who introduced me to the literature of systems theory. In the distant past, Paul David gave me a liberal education, John McCoy and others in the Department of Biostatistics and Epidemiology at the University of Oklahoma Health Sciences Center taught me professionalism, and Jack Sherry gave me a chance.

Los Altos, California   Karen A. Duncan
March 1994

The Author

Karen A. Duncan is a consultant to management on information systems in health care. She earned her B.S. degree (1964) in medical technology at the University of Oklahoma and both her M.S. degree (1968) and her Ph.D. degree (1970) in biostatistics at the University of Oklahoma Health Sciences Center. Duncan served on the faculty of the Medical University of South Carolina in Charleston and on the technical staff of the Mitre Corporation in McLean, Virginia, before starting her consulting practice in Los Altos, California, in 1980.

Duncan's research interests are in concepts of large-scale integrated information systems for health care and especially in creating the societal and professional framework within which such systems can be developed. She is the author or editor of numerous papers, reports, and books, including *A Model Curriculum for Doctoral-Level Programs in Health Computing* (1981, with R. H. Austing, S. Katz, R. E. Pengov, R. H. Pogue, and A. I. Wasserman) and *A History of Medical Informatics* (1990, with B. I. Blum). She is active in the International Federation for Information Processing and the Association for Computing Machinery and is a member of the American Medical Informatics Association, the Health Care Information and Management Systems Society, and the Association for Health Services Research.

Health Information
and Health Reform

PART ONE

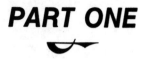

The Complexities of the System

Chapter One

A Crisis of Mission

Yes, the American health care system is in crisis. But this is not just a crisis of spiraling costs or administrative inefficiencies or crippling malpractice insurance premiums. These are pervasive problems that are symptoms of the crisis rather than the crisis itself. The real crisis goes much deeper: it goes to the heart of how health care is delivered, that is, to the caregiver-consumer relationship.

Both individually and collectively, health care providers have remained detached from recent debates about health care reform, in part because they do not see that the debates involve the crucial provider activities of patient care. Because the next steps in reform will have a powerful transforming impact on providers of care, however, their participation and leadership are essential.

Underlying Crises

The crisis in health care today is first and foremost a *crisis of mission.* It is evidenced by confusion about the values

3

and goals of caregivers and care receivers and of the values and goals of the institutions that support the unspoken compact between the system and the consumers of health care.

The crisis in health care is also to a large extent a *crisis of expectation,* that is, a crisis between the expectations of consumers of health care and the capabilities and intentions of the diverse elements of the health care delivery system. Finally, it is a *crisis of the unmet responsibilities* of each party to the compact. This aspect of the health care crisis came about because neither the health care system nor the people it serves have taken into account and acted on the changing circumstances of both the system and its environment. For instance, new considerations such as an aging population have largely been ignored by the system, and promising new tools such as information systems and techniques for quality improvement are being adopted too slowly.

One has only to listen to the concerns of the various stakeholders in health care to understand that each of these underlying crises has substance.

Stakeholders' Concerns

The stakeholders in health care are those who have a legitimate interest in its successful functioning; they are the patients, caregivers, institutions, suppliers, and payers. The following popular impressions of their diverse concerns are drawn collectively from newspaper and magazine accounts; they illustrate the disunity of stakeholders' perceptions of the mission of health care, their expectations

4

of the system, and their own and other stakeholders' responsibilities.

- Patients worry that they will be unable to get the medical care they may need in the future for myriad reasons. They worry that their insurance premiums will be unaffordable, that their insurance plan will drop them, that their company-paid plan choices won't cover what they need, that they will be forced to go to a doctor they do not like, or that they will be denied care. They worry about how they will pay for drugs, for long-term care, or for alternative care. They worry about whether they will be able to die with dignity. They do not know where to turn for information about the health care system or about their specific medical problems, and many do not even know where to go to get care.

- Physicians worry about loss of autonomy in selecting, treating, and charging patients. They worry about protecting their income, keeping up with the latest medical information, being sued, and having enough patients and a good relationship with their patients.

- Nurses know that they have the skills to do a great deal more for patients than they are allowed to do in such areas as case management and follow-up care. Moreover, they worry about being replaced in their current positions by less skilled and less expensive personnel.

- Health system workers, especially those who experience firsthand the extent of the clerical workload, worry about losing their jobs under administrative reform.

• Government agencies' staffs worry about how they are going to pay for what they have already promised, and they worry about fraud and waste. Elected officials worry about what citizens really want in the way of health care.

• Payers worry about regulation, the bottom line, and the elimination or transformation of their industry.

• Manufacturers worry about the cost of research, FDA approvals, price controls, regulation, and the bottom line.

• The business community worries about the increasingly large share of its revenues going to health care.

Significantly, issues affecting society as a whole, such as quality of care, the specter of rationing, and even such popular issues as access and cost, along with myriad ethical questions, do not appear to be the primary concern of any health care stakeholders. In general, the health care system is believed to be in crisis primarily because of its highly visible problems. But when critical systemwide, mission-oriented issues do not have a stakeholder constituency within the health care system, the crisis must have much deeper roots than previously supposed.

Deep Dissonances

The hallmark of a system in crisis is *dissonance,* and the health care system is no exception. Dissonances abound in the system, creating stresses and tensions among virtually all its elements. The immediacy of and disparity among stakeholders' perceptions and concerns dramatize the dissonance within the system, but there are even more serious things to worry about. Consider the following areas in which intractable and worsening circumstances seem to be outside the primary concerns of any stakeholder group.

Expanding Consumer Expectations

The gulf is vast between the educational preparation of health system workers and the health care needs of the nation. Medical training is centered on individual patients, and doctors are trained to provide diagnosis and treatment for their patients' specific medical problems. Virtually all health care personnel are trained, and facilities are organized, to support the doctor's role as provider of acute medical care to sick people.

Yet consumers need much more from the health care system than doctors who are trained to treat acute medical problems. They also need a way to obtain health education, preventive care, motivation, compliance, and chronic and long-term care, none of which are provided adequately if at all by the current system.

7

Shortage of Primary Caregivers

The widely acknowledged shortage of primary caregivers, especially in rural areas and inner cities, will be exacerbated if and when the millions of Americans who do not now have access to primary care are added to the system. However, a systemwide mechanism for dealing with this serious problem does not exist.

Advanced-Practice Nurses

Consumers would welcome nurse practitioners, and physician's assistants as well, as primary caregivers. However, except in unusual circumstances, these individuals are required to work under the supervision of a physician.

Medical Education

Even within the acute-care system, medical education is not providing the kinds of information that graduating physicians need. Each medical school develops its own curriculum; there is no systemwide mechanism for deciding what medical students need to know.

Medical Information Explosion

Consumers expect there to be mechanisms within the health care delivery system whereby their doctors keep up with new information and incorporate it into their practices. In fact, doctors are losing the race to keep pace with new knowledge and new technologies.

Resources for Outcomes Research

In a relatively new area of health services research called outcomes research, several government and professional groups are searching the medical literature for information that can be used to develop definitive guidelines for treatment in selected major diagnoses where current treatment patterns are significantly diverse.

Surprisingly, an exhaustive examination of the literature has thus far shown that many studies are flawed and cannot be used collectively to establish guidelines. Expensive and time-consuming clinical trials will be needed; in the meantime, physicians are practicing without this guidance.

Research Priorities

In medical research, funding priorities are set with seeming disregard for society's needs and values. Consumers have only recently become aware of this through publicity about the inequitable quantity of research on AIDS and on certain diseases in women.

Health Information Bottleneck

Public health information that consumers need in order to take responsibility for their health and health care is available piecemeal or not at all and typically from unofficial sources. It is seldom in a form that is useful.

Ethical Concerns

Ethical questions raised by the use of new health care technologies, especially at the beginning and end of life, are addressed only locally, if at all. The social implications are far-reaching, and the absence of meaningful guidance for providers and consumers causes great unnecessary pain.

Profit Motive

Health care has been perceived traditionally as a profession in which the practitioners are motivated more by altruism than by profit. However, many medical businesses such as laboratories, claim-processing agencies, and pharmaceutical companies appear to be primarily profit oriented. Even managed-care organizations, the very names of which have been synonymous with fiscal prudence in the past, such as Blue Cross of California, are moving increasingly into the for-profit sector.

Lack of National Policy

Consumers expect and believe that medical professional groups such as the American Medical Association, in concert with public agencies such as those of the United States Department of Health and Human Services, have a responsibility for determining and enforcing health policy. However, health care providers know that there is no unifying health policy in the United States, no effective policy-making body for any segment—or the whole—of the health care system, and no agreed-upon set of principles that guide the decisions of individual providers.

The foregoing examples serve to show the deep dissonances that exist in the health care system. They cut across the immediate concerns of the various stakeholder groups and reflect dissonance in perceptions of *mission,* dissonance in the groups' *expectations,* and dissonance in the sense of *responsibility* that the various stakeholders feel toward health care.

It is not enough, however, simply to identify the kinds of crises and dissonances plaguing the health care system. Before effective solutions can be proposed, it is necessary to understand the underlying causes and the forces at work that have brought them about.

Confronting Complexity

It is only reasonable that the collective problems within a system as complex as the health care system would seem to be overwhelming and intractable. The system is complex in many ways.

- Its sheer size and scope make it complex. About 8.5 million people work in the health care system. Its budget is bigger than that of most countries, and it reaches into every corner of the United States, affecting almost every aspect of society.
- It has a rich diversity of stakeholders, functions, and interests.
- It is culturally and sociologically diverse and complex, both internally and in its interactions with the rest of society.
- It has a rigid and entrenched structure and approach to doing business that are very difficult to change.

Of course, complexity makes problem solving very difficult, but it can be made easier by confronting complexity systematically by trying to understand the root causes of problems and then using this information to develop and assess solutions. Such an approach—a *systems approach*—requires first developing an understanding of the system in its entirety, including its values, scope, functions, nature, history, evolution, and impact on and relationship with its environment and other systems.

This approach can be likened to peeling back the layers of an onion and then reassembling them correctly. Reassembly can recapture all the original complexity only if the process of disassembly produces an understanding of the onion as a system. Solutions offered will then follow from an analysis based on that understanding.

Traditionally, decision makers do not use a systems approach, at least in part because only recently in our history has it become evident that our problems are so complex that a systems approach is needed to understand and solve them. This realization has come particularly late to solvers of socially based problems such as those of the health care system, if indeed it has come at all. Policy makers and other decision makers tend, naturally and/or by lack of training, to focus on those portions of complex problems that they believe they understand and for which they have solutions. In effect, they ignore complexity.

Examples abound in health care. Health care reform debaters focus almost exclusively on the organization and financing of health care, apparently in the mistaken belief that the science of health care—physician decisions about patients—is well established and can be ignored as a factor in cost containment. They similarly ignore the complex sociology of the system, perhaps in the hope that intangible elements such as caregiver-patient relationships and ethical issues such as rationing will automatically adjust to organizational changes. Most seriously of all, reform debaters do not seem to realize the scale of unintended consequences likely to occur when one tries to impose radical change on the structure and function of one-seventh of the nation's economy. In human terms, this is on the same scale as trying to move the location of your leg on your body and change its function. Although health care is primarily a conceptual system and your body is a physical system, the extent of disruption is probably comparable.

The most careful analysis humanly possible is called for. As already noted, however, it is not enough just to study the problems. In Part One of this book, we take the classical systems approach of examining relevant aspects of the entire system in order to decide what the underlying causes of crises and problems are before looking for solutions. That is, we try systematically to understand how the stakeholders' diverse concerns have developed and why such deep dissonances as those between consumer and caregiver needs and system capabilities have come about.

Approaching Solutions

Following the analysis, the underlying causes of dissonance in the health care system are shown to fall into three areas. First, the system, which is larger than most countries, *does not have an infrastructure* within which it can govern itself. It needs a legislative body to set policy and an executive body to carry it out. Second, as problems have developed, the health care system apparently *has been unable or unwilling to take the lead* in their solution; the federal government has stepped into the vacuum. Third, caregivers, consumers, educators, researchers, and policy makers *do not have the information they need* for the effective function of the system to deliver health care. Much of the information needed to bring the system to a state where it can serve well into the next century exists but is unavailable. The system suffers from a severe blockage of information flow that is hampering achievement of the potential of modern medical and communications technology.

Information that could be used for health education, research, clinical decision making, and policy formation is trapped almost at its origins. It is trapped in research laboratories, textbooks, and journals, and it is trapped in patient records in the back rooms of clinics and the basements of hospitals. Information is also trapped in the files of third-party payers and in the minds of providers and consumers. As a result, it is simply inaccessible to those who might be guided by its collective wisdom.

Operationally, the tools exist to deliver information where it is needed and to assist in the effective use of information. However, the health care system has not yet taken full advantage of these tools, which are methodological (such as biostatistics), managerial (such as practice management techniques), and technological (such as computer systems).

The underlying causes of infrastructural, leadership, and information flow problems are systemwide and national in scope, and their solutions must be so as well. The problems are so extensive and pervasive that it only makes economic sense (the systems approach again) to find solutions on a national basis. In the absence of national leadership from within the system, stakeholders have grown accustomed to implementing piecemeal solutions, where each stakeholder group or geographic region devises its own disconnected solutions. This approach further exacerbates dissonance as, for instance, small and large groups of providers band together to set their own competitive prices and standards for care.

The problems in our system and their underlying causes affect all stakeholders, and because of the magnitude of the problems, all stakeholders are affected regardless of whether solutions are designed piecemeal or devised for the benefit of the entire system. A systems approach therefore requires that all stakeholders collaborate in designing the solutions. This will not be easy for a system that has no infrastructure and is unaccustomed to providing leadership for solving its own problems. Yet because the dissonances of unmet informational needs are shown in this book to be primarily in clinical arenas, it is essential that the health care system take the lead.

The Role of Information Technology

We are fortunate to be living in the information age at the very time when our social problems are so complex as to need the help of information technology—computers and communications technology—to understand and solve them. Solutions to information-based problems such as those caused by lack of good information fortunately can be facilitated with information technology. In fact, in this case they cannot be solved without information technology. The technology can also facilitate the establishment of an infrastructure and help leaders lead. We propose a National Health Information System (NHIS) for precisely those purposes.

The NHIS ideas are not introduced until Part Two of the book, however, to underscore the importance of first performing the analysis and assessment from which the solution will flow. Although the proposed NHIS would be based on a computer and telecommunications network, the discussion is not technical; rather, it focuses on the conceptual design of the network and how it would function to benefit the health care system.

Defining the Limits of Concern

Given the complexity of the health care system and the extent of the crisis, proposing a solution for every problem would be beyond the scope of this or any other book. The focus here is on those problems that seem intractable without the use of information technology. Fortunately, the systems approach can be applied by others to problems not adequately addressed here, including problems such as commitment to quality improvement, for which information technology is not the primary solution.

Because the proposed NHIS is indeed national in scope, with telecommunications linkages to regional and local information systems, readers who work with institutional applications of information technology will recognize the essential role they would play in NHIS-based solutions. However, because institutionally based applications are widely described elsewhere, we acknowledge their importance but do not discuss them further, except as they relate to the national system.

For two other classes of problems in health care, we identify the problem but do not analyze them. These are (1) problems whose solutions seem so straightforward and reasonable in their *common sense* that one wonders why they are debated at all and (2) issues that relate to society's notions of *ethics or morality.* Some of these would benefit from the use of information technology, but they do not need to wait for the NHIS to begin their solution.

In terms of common sense, some changes that need to be made in the health care system are obvious and not sufficiently complex to warrant further equivocating. When these changes are made, the winners will be both the health care system and the American people. These include reducing administrative waste due to incompatible billing systems, initiating insurance reform so that all who want and need coverage can get it, and selecting payment systems based on considerations of cost and efficiency.

In terms of ethics, society's values should be the driving force behind reform choices in several areas of health care. Included here are issues surrounding the beginning and end of life, such as whether to treat extremely premature infants or those with severe medical problems (Young, 1989); issues associated with the potential rationing of

17

health care to achieve broader access to care; issues surrounding the use of quality of life indicators as a factor in treatment planning; and the issue of using health care dollars to provide large profits for some stakeholders.

Although this book discusses *what* needs to be done, it stops short of discussing *how* it should be done. The vast organizational, sociological, political, and technological problems are real and will be difficult to overcome; nonetheless, they must be overcome. Further, it is clear from the analysis just *who* should do it—the health care system. Readers are invited to consider as they follow the analysis and solutions whether there is any other group equipped to define, design, and implement the proposed National Health Information System.

Finally, the systems approach requires us not only to solve existing problems but also to create a goal-directed health care system that avoids such problems in the future. Therefore, Part Three of this book envisions an NHIS that will not only serve the needs we can foresee today but will also serve as a transforming agent that will enable the health care system to fulfill its mission at last.

Chapter Two

A Systematic Appraisal

The mission of a social system such as health care is to fulfill specific needs of the society it serves. In that context the *values* of our society should determine the kind of health care system we need. They should shape the *mission* of the system and give focus to its *goals*. So we begin at the beginning with a consideration of those guiding values.

Values for Health Care

Priester (1992, p. 85) believes that frustrations with health care arise from deep "disagreement and confusion about the values that should shape America's health care system." He suggests the need for explicit values for health care to guide reform efforts. Americans are so unaccustomed to thinking about social values with respect to health care that many ethical/moral issues are not even recognized as such. Instead, as we shall see, they frequently masquerade as practical problems.

In past decades when health care was much simpler and not always available, diverse values were not really relevant. The doctor-patient relationship was truly the business of only the doctor and the patient, and there were very few choices to be made. Today, however, the selective availability and relative high cost of life-saving high technology, combined with the intrusive authority of those who hold medicine's purse strings, are forcing us to examine for the first time our social values relative to health care.

Because its social traditions are rooted in notions of individual freedom and autonomy, the United States often finds its traditional social institutions in conflict with its awakening consciousness of universal humanity. Elsewhere in the industrial world, this consciousness has already led to widespread development of social support systems such as universal health care. Those in the United States who advocate access to health care for all people have portrayed our health care system as being socially unevolved. But is this the case, or does our current system in fact reflect the values of the American people?

Whether health care is a privilege or a right is an issue fraught with provocative undercurrents. While current reform efforts assume that universal access to some level of health care is an American value, such a belief has not guided the system in the past. This unresolved question of right versus privilege and its logical extensions underlie all of contemporary reform debate. Let us ask—but not answer—the following questions right now.

Is health care a right or a privilege?

If it is a right, is it a right, like voting, that is up to the individual to exercise?

If it is a right, how much health care does this mean?

Should anyone be able to get whatever they need, regardless of the cost?

Who is to decide what a person needs?

Would the same rules apply no matter what a person's age or health status, for example, a newborn or a terminally ill individual?

Sometimes practical concerns such as a lack of transportation prevent a person from seeing a doctor. Should solving such ancillary problems of access be a part of health care?

These kinds of questions highlight the conflicting social goals that result from the diverse values held by Americans. Here are some health care system manifestations of those conflicting social goals. Too often, "cost" is a surrogate concern that allows us to avoid many value-oriented issues.

Price controls versus free enterprise: Health care businesses should be like any other, but if we do not control prices, we may not be able to have health care for everyone.

Access versus cost: Everyone should have health care, but we cannot afford to pay for it all.

Choice versus cost: People want to be able to change doctors freely, but free-choice plans are too expensive.

Patient autonomy versus cost: If a doctor and patient decide on a particular course of treatment, plan administrators should not be able to deny payment; if a patient wants to see a specialist, a gatekeeper should not be able to deny referral.

Quality of care versus cost: Development of practice guidelines and medical decision aids is very time-consuming and expensive.

Quality of care versus human relationships: Practice guidelines and medical decision aids might improve quality of care, but they also might depersonalize care.

Quality of life versus cost: Is it really medical care if the benefits are primarily subjective—that is, primarily a matter of the patient "feeling" better, for instance?

Impulse for life versus quality of life: The sanctity of life is weighed against the notions of a life worth living—a consideration when a baby will be born with severe defects, for instance.

Individual versus collective health care: Individuals want the best possible care for themselves and their families, but they are not entirely comfortable with offering the same care to their neighbors, even though the value of a healthy populace is clear.

It is important to understand that these are truly matters of value and not mere practicality. To illustrate, if these really were questions of practicality, then guidelines for the medical care of 750-gram newborn babies or seriously ill elderly people would be cost and resource based (rationing). Instead, we have at best a hodgepodge of guidelines that vary from institution to institution and case to case. Clearly, values are at stake. Whether we can deliver the care and whether and how it should be paid for should be secondary to the question of whether or not our society places value on, and *has as a goal,* the delivery of such care. That is, it is appropriate that goals of social systems should have ethical rather than practical foundations.

Regardless of whether the health care system met society's needs in the past, it is now clear that society and the system have evolved in different ways and need to be reconciled. Thus the analysis should point toward solutions that include mechanisms whereby society can understand the nature of health care issues and resolve those in its realm of responsibility.

General System Characteristics

A system can exist in many dimensions, each of which has its own parameters. Health care has at least physical, functional, social, and conceptual dimensions. Physically, it is composed of facilities, agents, and tools. Its functions relate primarily to patient care and its many supporting processes. Socially, it is composed of networks and hierarchies of people and their interactions. The dimension of primary interest in this book is the conceptual one because we are dealing with ideas about what the health care system could be and because our objective is to establish conceptual frameworks within which the future system can evolve.

In this context, the health care system is composed of our notions of health and illness, the rules by which we maintain health and cure illness, and the infrastructure that supports the system, including notions of education, research, credentialing, quality assurance, policy, and ethics.

Keeping these factors in mind, we next consider whether the health care system is a "good" system in the sense that it has all the elements and characteristics a system needs to function and meet its goals. A body of work called general systems theory identifies these kinds of characteristics, which we will examine before applying them to health care.

Goals: Good systems are clear about what their goals are. The focus of activities within good systems is toward those goals.

Subsystems: The subsystems, or elements, of a good system are clear about their roles in the system. The goals of the subsystems are congruent with the goals of the system as a whole, and activities of the subsystems are focused on their respective goals and on the goals of the system.

Hierarchy: A good system must have a hierarchy that is adequate to manage its complexity.

Boundaries: In a good system, the boundaries between the system and its environment and between the system and its subsystems are clear; further, the boundaries between the subsystems are clear.

Resources: A good system's resources are adequate and are distributed effectively throughout the system.

Functions: All functions that the system needs to reach its goals are carried out effectively by the system and its appropriate subsystems. Moreover, all major functions of the system are goal directed.

Interaction: In a good subsystem communication is open between the system and the environment and among all subsystems.

Inputs: A good system uses the inputs it receives effectively and continuously.

Outputs: A good system produces outputs consistent with its goals.

Feedback: A good system accepts and acts on feedback from its environment, from other systems on its level, and from its subsystems.

Equifinality: A good system allows for more than one acceptable way of reaching its goals.

The purpose of applying these characteristics to health care is not to judge but to identify areas where constructive change is needed.

Analysis of the Health Care System

Reform efforts need to be firmly rooted in system goals that reflect our society's values, but just what those goals

25

should be is not an issue that can be resolved here. We have therefore arbitrarily selected the following mission statement for health care that can be used to derive goals: *The mission of the health care system is to promote good health for all Americans and to restore their health in case of need.*

Goals

Now we can state the following general goals, which we will need in order to continue the analysis.

- Good health and health care should be available to everyone.
- Health care should be of the best possible quality.
- Health care should be affordable.

Practical considerations may prevent us from fully achieving these goals, but we still must plan and strive. Now that we have a set of goals for guidance, we can see how the present health care system measures up.

It has already been noted that, for whatever reasons, the health care system seems to have lost sight of society's expectations. Increasing numbers of people do not have access to health care, the quality of health care is largely unassessed, and health care is becoming less and less affordable. To the extent that the foregoing goals are acceptable, the system is falling behind, with no remedies of its own in sight.

Subsystems

The primary subsystems, or elements, of the health care system are the providers and consumers of health care.

Throughout this book, the term *providers* refers to all caregivers, including but not limited to hospitals, physicians, and nurses. However, the health care system cannot function without an extensive array of supporting subsystems—its functional infrastructure. Some of these are administrative structures, third-party payers, manufacturers and suppliers, and libraries. Still other important supporting subsystems are the conceptual ones of research, education, professional associations, credentialing and certification, quality assurance, planning, and policy-making.

The functional elements of the health care system also happen to be its stakeholders. Throughout this book, the term *element* is used in functional contexts, and the word *stakeholder* is used in all other contexts. While an analysis of individual stakeholders' commitment to the mission of the system is beyond the scope of this book, we can consider their collective commitment to system goals and their role in achieving them.

All stakeholders probably agree that quality of care is important, but no particular stakeholder is charged with responsibility for the quality of care, nor is this a major component of the activities of most stakeholders, individually or collectively.

All stakeholders probably agree that access to health care is important, but no particular stakeholder is responsible for ensuring reasonable access, nor is this a component of the activities of most stakeholders, individually or collectively.

All stakeholders probably agree that cost containment is very important, but no stakeholder or group of stakeholders is specifically responsible for cost containment.

The system is preoccupied with illness rather than health. No element is responsible for keeping people healthy. As a practical matter, the system seems to have disowned health and has even suggested that consumers take over the responsibility for it.

It appears that the system is made up of whatever it is that its subsystems do rather than of subsystems whose mission it is to work together to serve the goals of the system. The picture is one of a system without substance; it seems to be no more than the sum of its parts.

Boundaries

The boundaries between the system and its environment—the society it serves—have traditionally been so well defined that almost no one outside the system has really understood or tried to look at what it has done to carry out its mission. Now the boundaries are less clear; outside groups have usurped some of the functions of the health care system, such as the promotion of public health and health policy formation. On the other hand, the boundaries between the system and its stakeholders and also between stakeholders are still so clearly defined that little communication seems to take place beyond the operational level. That is, provider groups do not work toward the system mission together or with other stakeholders such as insurance companies or consumers.

Resources

It is difficult to determine whether the system's resources are really adequate because they are so inequitably distributed. For instance, many geographic areas have an excess of providers while others have almost none. Other indicators of inequitable distribution are the extent of excessive and inappropriate use of technology, uneven access, skewed research priorities, and the extent of resources used to generate large profits.

Hierarchy

The system has reached a level of complexity that is beyond its control; it does not have the hierarchy it needs to cope. There is no system infrastructure that would bring stakeholders together for cooperative, mission-oriented action (Shannon, 1983).

Functions

Several key goal-directed functions such as maintaining health do not seem to have a place in the health care system. In fact, the system appears to revolve around *activities* rather than *functions*. Activities might be "treat the sick," "send the bill," "publish the research." While these are of course essential activities, it is not clear that a sufficient proportion of the system's activities are part of goal-directed functions.

Further, the system is in danger of having a significant portion of its resources diverted to serve goals other than its own. Consider whether the federal effort to balance the budget on the back of the health care system is a function that serves health care goals.

Interaction

Communication beyond that needed for specific operational activities is rare among stakeholders. That is, communication appears to be mostly for the purpose of passing patients through the system and not for the purpose of interacting to develop approaches to mission fulfillment. A notable exception is the cooperative effort among many professional groups to encourage the development of a computer-based patient record.

Inputs and Outputs

Inputs to the system are consumers in search of good health, which they expect to find within the health care system.

Outputs of the system, as compared to goals, fall short:

All elements of the health care system are geared toward treating disease, not toward maintaining or improving health.

With respect to quality, American health care is generally considered by Americans to be the best, even though many nations rank higher than the United States on such indicators as infant mortality, immunization rates, and longevity. Recent indications are that quality of output will be further called into question as the extent of the inappropriate use of technology becomes clear.

Affordability of patient care is also not acceptable.

Feedback

Society has been very vocal about such major problems as cost, quality, and equity, but the health care system has not yet been responsive. Rather than proactively tackling these problems as a system, each stakeholder group has taken the path of adjusting in its own fashion to the edicts of payers and policy makers who are attempting to find their own solutions.

Equifinality

Several different approaches to mission fulfillment are possible. We cannot take comfort in this, however, because any selected approach or combination of approaches must stand up to the same criteria of a good system. For example, organizational and financing reforms can only have the desired effect if they are carried out in the context of the mission of health care. That is, they must address such missing functions as provision for health maintenance and quality assurance as well as cost control and improved access. Without such comprehensive reforms, the current system will simply assimilate and adjust to administrative changes as it has done for the past thirty years, its fundamental flaws unaddressed and uncured.

Gaps in the System

We have seen that the health care system lacks many of the characteristics of a good system. The most critical shortcomings are:

- The system does not work toward goals that are based on society's values and needs.
- Many critical functions such as health maintenance are not being carried out.
- Resources are distributed inequitably.
- The system lacks the level of hierarchy—the conceptual infrastructure—that is needed to carry out overall planning and coordination of goal-driven functions.

As was the case in the discussion of values, our analysis should later point to solutions that include supplying these mission-essential characteristics.

Chapter Three

The Demand for Change

As individuals, we know how to control our costs and distribute our resources to cover our highest priorities, so it seems reasonable to doubt that self-management in health care could be as bad as it appears to be. Such doubt can lead to proposals for simplistic solutions to problems that are in fact due to underlying forces that have become deeply ingrained over a period of fifty years. For instance, a remedy once suggested for problems of physician distribution was to change physicians' incentives by increasing the number of physicians. But we shall see how this only exacerbated the problems it was intended to solve. The reality is that many aspects of the current crisis are symptoms of even deeper dissonances, so attempts to correct them without addressing the underlying forces will only create more dissonance.

In this chapter we further peel back the onion of complexity by looking at the forces at work in the health care system as it has evolved over the past fifty years. We then predict how the health care system will continue to evolve over the next several years, if these forces are not mitigated. To some extent, the health care system has developed in response to the same forces that have operated on the rest of society. For example, our post–World War II affluence, the cycle of inflation and recession, and the political agenda of the party in power certainly have had an effect. Nevertheless, to a surprising degree, the health care system is the victim of its own internal machinations.

What follows is not intended to be a history of health care; rather, it provides information that will help explain a *point of view* about the modern evolution of the health care system. That point of view reveals an increasingly discordant system that is the victim of its own successes and prosperity, its failure to manage, and its unwillingness to lead. Evolution has a past and a future, and we shall look at both in this chapter. The past must be examined for clues to the present, so we begin with a snapshot of health care nearly fifty years ago.

The Post–World War II Climate

Following World War II, the foundations of modern health care were well established (Starr, 1982). Hard-won physician sovereignty prevailed in matters involving medical decision making, and most health care was delivered in individual doctors' offices. The National Institutes of Health was in place, and medical research had become a national priority; the scientific basis for health care was improving. Formal medical education stopped with an internship, but doctors kept up with new developments by reading and attending medical society meetings.

The lines between public health and medicine were clearly drawn, with public health having relatively low status. Hospitals were nonprofit entities, and administrative control of hospitals was well established. Between the doctors and the hospitals, a substantial amount of free medical care was given. Blue Cross and Blue Shield and private insurance were available, and employer payment of premiums was common. Health care was a privilege, not necessarily a right.

The Beginnings of Change

The next twenty-five years were a period of prosperity for health care as growth occurred throughout the system. Medical schools were booming because of expanded research funding; the increasing amount of medical knowledge required longer periods of medical education, which abetted the formation of medical specialties. To cope with the volume of new publications, in 1965 the National Library of Medicine (NLM) automated its catalogue indexing system, MEDLARS. To bring the new research findings to specialists and other health care practitioners, researchers, and educators, in 1971 the NLM began making its catalogues available at remote computer terminals through a system called MEDLINE.

Further support for increasing the number of specialists came from government subsidies for specialist training and higher insurance payments to specialists. The benefits of specialist residency programs to the sponsoring hospitals were also a factor in increasing the number of specialists because the system of specialist certification in effect did not provide for regulation of the number or distribution of specialties.

At the same time, concerns for broader access to care led to several attempts at the federal level to legislate public funding for universal health care. Largely through the influence of the American Medical Association (AMA), these efforts were deflected into programs that would "improve" health care by improving selected specific subsystems of health care. Here are some examples of the narrow focus, all of which were accomplished by grant mechanisms, thus avoiding government control of the programs.

The Hill-Burton program of 1946, which sought to improve access to care in low-income states, supported extensive building of new hospitals.

The Regional Medical Program of 1965 set up regional networks that integrated research, education, and medical care for heart disease, cancer, and stroke.

The Medicare and Medicaid programs were launched in 1965 to pay for medical care of the aged and to help support the states' care for the poor.

Neighborhood and community health centers were established in the mid-1960s, primarily by the Department of Health, Education, and Welfare (now Health and Human Services) and the Office of Economic Opportunity, to provide coordinated ambulatory care services of all types in low-income areas.

The Health Manpower Act of 1971 paid medical schools to increase their enrollments in the hope that new physicians would establish practices in underserved areas.

Cost Concerns Begin to Dominate

By the early 1970s, in our greatly expanded and prosperous system of health care, the "mandate ran out. The economic and moral problems of medicine displaced scientific progress at the center of public attention. . . . American medicine seemed to pass from stubborn shortages to irrepressible excess, without ever having passed through happy sufficiency" (Starr, 1982, p. 379). Health care's excessive command of national resources was beginning to be felt, and the system was generally considered to be in crisis. The government's major stake in health care spending, primarily through the Medicare and Medicaid programs, gave impetus to its deeper involvement.

One significant precedent set during this period was the 1972 establishment of Professional Standards Review Organizations (PSROs) to ensure that Medicare patients, whose care was being paid for by the federal government, were treated appropriately. Although only physicians could make judgments about care on behalf of the PSROs, and although no national standards were imposed, for the first time the government had given hospitals a means to control the clinical decisions of physicians. Medicare would not pay hospitals for physician care it deemed inappropriate.

The door to government involvement in clinical practice had been opened.

Another important move in this period was the beginning of federal support for the Health Maintenance Organization (HMO) concept, which is the use of prepaid group practice to control costs and reverse the incentives that rewarded doctors and hospitals for treating illness instead of maintaining health. Although these organizations did not grow at the rate originally envisioned—HMOs were to have been available to 90 percent of the population by 1980—they did become an increasingly significant factor in the future of health care.

In 1974, advocates of systemwide planning were encouraged by the National Health Planning and Resource Development Act, which established a system of agencies from the national to the local level for health planning and implementation. The centerpiece was two hundred regional Health Systems Agencies (HSAs) that would include consumer representatives. The aim was to contain costs through control of capital expenditures and to improve access to care within a region by planning for needed facilities and staff. Although the underfunded and underpowered HSAs had little impact while they were in existence, they serve to highlight the significant absence of such planning groups today.

Second only to concerns for cost were the continuing concerns for access. Surprisingly, even in that era of increasing government involvement, access issues continued to be addressed piecemeal.

The Window of Opportunity Begins to Close

Despite increasing systemwide complexity and outside pressures during the 1970s (primarily the threat of competition from the congressionally mandated HMOs and the prospect of increasing government control), no overarching organization encompassing physicians, hospitals, insurance companies, and other stakeholders had been developed within the health care system to take charge of shaping its future service to the American people. A public health role had long been abdicated by physicians, but organized public health such as the federal Public Health Service had little clout or role in the system, and public health interests simply were not a factor in trying to organize the complex, overweight system.

Physician organizations and others within the system continued to react to outside initiatives rather than become proactive in facing the problems of health care. Further, with the rising power and divergent interests of the academic-research side of medicine, the cohesiveness of physicians in general was eroding. Those aspects of the health care system that still sustained physician sovereignty were respect for their scholarly professionalism, concerns for patient privacy, and the fact that few people outside the medical profession really understood what health care was all about.

Cost Control with a Vengeance

Although concern for rising health care costs had reached the level of alarm, there were really no mechanisms within

39

the health care system by which cost control could even be attempted. Attempts to do so were largely voluntary until 1984, when the Health Care Financing Administration (HCFA) introduced prospective payment to hospitals for Medicare patients on a case-by-case basis. HCFA was able to establish prospective payment because it had access to the enormous database of patient information that it had collected in the course of reimbursing hospitals for the care of Medicare patients. Information in the database was used to develop a set of Diagnosis-Related Groups (DRGs). A fixed amount of money (with adjustments) would be paid to a hospital for the stay of any given patient whose illness fell into a specific DRG.

The theory was that efficiently managed hospitals would find payments based on DRGs adequate; however, few hospitals found this to be the case. Although the introduction of DRGs did reduce costs to the Medicare program for a few years, it had several other impacts. Over the next ten years, 10 percent of all private hospitals closed their doors. The natural response of hospitals that did not close was to keep their operating budgets in the black by billing their privately insured patients for the difference between their costs and their reimbursements, a practice known as cost shifting. A further consequence of DRGs was "DRG creep," the practice of assigning a patient to the highest-paying DRG that could be justified.

Hospitals were also facing pressure from insurance companies, which required that more and more procedures be done on an outpatient basis, where they could usually be done at less cost. At the same time, unaffiliated hospitals faced competition with HMOs, which were drawing increasing numbers of patients off the market. Hospital bed occupancy rates were falling and so were revenues. Hospitals responded by opening or expanding their own outpatient centers, offering new services, or affiliating themselves with other providers to offer a broader range of health services. Health care marketing was key, and hospitals and integrated groups of all kinds competed for the health care dollar. While various segments benefited in the short term, none of these activities could be considered to be cost control measures for the system as a whole.

The 1980s were also a time of heightened activity in the business community, as corporate pricing and profits were threatened by escalating health care costs. Many businesses banded together in regional groups to search for solutions. Some companies instituted wellness programs to keep their employees healthy. To control administrative costs, some very large companies self-insured. Most began to offer a variety of health plans, including the required HMO option, that were designed to encourage employees to take some responsibility for holding down costs. Increasingly, employees were seeing only physicians who were part of an approved, less expensive plan.

In the physician community, a serious shortage of primary care doctors was developing. Many new graduates opted to go directly into a prepaid practice rather than face the uncertainties of setting up their own practice in the current climate. To ensure an adequate patient base, physicians in private practice joined a variety of plans in record numbers. HMOs and other prepaid plans were on the rise. Ancillary primary care providers such as midwives and nurse practitioners gained ground, and groups increasingly used nurses as "gatekeepers" into their practices.

Meanwhile in the insurance industry, both administrative costs and payments for health care were increasing. Insurance companies tried to control their own costs through such devices as requiring doctors to obtain pre-authorization for most hospitalizations and charging premiums according to the actual medical experiences (past or expected) of the individual or group (experience rating). They also refused coverage to increasing numbers of people with preexisting medical conditions that would have been covered in the past.

At the same time, the federal government continued its attempts to control its costs by increasing Medicare premiums and curbing its contributions to Medicaid, forcing the states either to pay a larger share of the cost of medical care for the poor or to institute rationing of health care. A number of states responded by instituting forms of rationing, either by revising eligibility requirements or by limiting what services they would cover.

The government's next large-scale attempt to control its own costs was aimed directly at physicians. Since care by nonspecialists is generally cheaper, HCFA reasoned that care that does not require delivery by a specialist should therefore be encouraged. Thus HCFA again used its Medicare database as a cost-cutting tool, this time to develop a scheme for reapportioning its payments to physicians so that more of the total funding would go for primary care. The Resource-Based Relative Value Scale (RBRVS) rates what doctors do according to several criteria and calculates reimbursement according to each procedure's score.

By the end of the 1980s, consumers began to realize that there was a serious problem with health care, and they made it second only to the economy as a 1992 election issue. They could see direct evidence of rising costs; the papers were full of stories about the growing numbers of uninsured, especially among the poor and children; and the specter of an AIDS epidemic dramatized the need for reform in the organization and prioritization of medical research.

Health services researchers began taking a very serious look at how other countries finance health care and found that not only is health care cheaper in all other industrialized countries but the United States is the only one without a national plan of paying for health care for all its citizens.

The 1980s were a decade of astonishing technological advances and of dizzying change in the health care system. However, although access improved for some groups, conditions worsened for many others. Also, despite the extensive concern for cost containment, little was accomplished.

Evolutionary and Compensatory Dissonance

Before examining the next stage in the evolutionary path of the health care system—the system as it is today—let's first consider how concepts of dissonance have been manifested in the system so far. Dissonance occurs when elements of a system work at cross-purposes to other elements, the system as a whole, and/or the system's environment. An escalating amount of intractable dissonance has become a striking feature of the health care system in recent years. Problems that have been recognized for many years, such as access, cost, and the proliferation of untested technology, have resisted solution. Too often what have appeared to be solutions have caused yet another set of problems. This is a clear signal that policy makers have not yet understood and acted upon the complexity of the underlying causes.

Compensatory dissonance occurs when one system element tries to compensate, in a way that is contrary to overall system goals, for the way that it was affected by changes made by another element. No value judgment is implied per se. For instance, compensatory dissonance occurred when hospitals responded to the imposition of DRGs by assigning the highest justifiable DRG in each case—DRG creep. The compensatory dissonance created in turn negated a part of the very cost savings that DRGs were supposed to achieve, an effect that was disruptive to both Medicare and the overall health care system.

A system can also show *evolutionary dissonance,* provided the adjustments it makes are a natural consequence of trying to meet the goals of the system. An example of evolutionary dissonance is the disruption caused by the introduction of information technology for a hospital record system.

Both compensatory dissonance and evolutionary dissonance are useful concepts for understanding why many problems in the health care system seem so intractable because both concepts help us consider whether changes and responses are proactive and goal-serving (evolutionary) or reactive and self-serving (compensatory). That is, dissonances that can be understood to occur in response to genuine system needs (such as care for an aging population) and opportunities for growth (new technologies) can be viewed as evolutionary cornerstones for the future health care system; dissonances that preserve the institutionalized status quo or self-interests of stakeholders without regard to system goals are compensatory and can be harmful to the system as a whole.

The rest of this section focuses on access, impact of medical research, and DRGs, areas in which the interplay of evolutionary and compensatory dissonance has become an increasingly significant factor in the evolution of the health care system. They illustrate how the compensatory dissonance that is shaping the system today has its roots in well-intentioned actions and reactions taken some forty years ago.

Early Evolution of Access

The nation was unable to satisfy its awakening social concern for access to health care in the period following World War II. Attempts to legislate universal access were blocked primarily by the efforts of the AMA. Since the federal government was unable to deal directly with access (by, for example, placing doctors where they were needed most), it dealt with access indirectly and piecemeal. For example, it helped fund the building of more hospitals in states that were underserved, gave medical schools the money to graduate more physicians, and created Medicare and Medicaid.

When these measures took full effect, access certainly improved for some segments of the patient population. However, the measures also had some natural side effects that were initially evolutionary but which later led to compensatory dissonances. Consider the following examples:

• When the new hospitals were built and more hospital beds became available, doctors put patients in them for medical conditions that previously did not require hospitalization, such as terminal illness and the delivery of babies. Overall system costs increased when the new services were introduced because of increased physician utilization and an increase in health service workers, goods, and supplies.

• When more physicians graduated from medical school, they established their practices in geographic areas that they believed could support them. Thus, new physicians tended to cluster around urban and suburban middle-class and affluent communities. The resulting surplus of physicians in these areas meant fewer patients per physician. To achieve and maintain their expected and needed income, physicians raised their fees and did more work per patient.

When Medicare and Medicaid were enacted, millions of people who had not had care before, or who had had only free care, began to receive care. Almost overnight health care became profitable, making it an attractive investment both for the business community and for physician-entrepreneurs. While this was good for doctors, hospitals, patients, suppliers, and investors, overall system costs rose rapidly.

Expanded Emphasis on Research

Medicine had been striving for decades to become more scientific, and research was a highly respected national priority following World War II. Most research was conducted at medical centers associated with medical schools, and expanding faculties devoted an increasing proportion of their time to the research that produced revenue for their institutions. As the base of medical knowledge expanded, so did the length of physician training, the number of kinds of specialties, and the number of specialists. The medical community began to polarize between community physicians and academic-research physicians. To this point the dissonance was primarily natural and evolutionary.

The physician community's preoccupation with science led to a decline in the status of primary care. Blessed with better general health and increasing personal mobility, the country almost lost sight of the concept of a personal family physician. Medical schools' attempts to place more emphasis on family practice were not effective in stemming the rush of graduates into specialties. Two compensatory dissonances were established here. First, an imbalance developed between generalists and specialists. Second, a generation of adults never learned to appreciate and value the services of a traditional family physician. The consequences for the system as a whole were not foreseen as each individual medical student, or even each teaching institution, made the decision to foster specialization.

The expansion of medical knowledge led inevitably to rapid development of profitable new medical technologies of every sort. The new technologies included laboratory and other types of tests; surgical and nonsurgical therapeutic procedures, devices, pharmaceuticals, and biotechnology products; and new processes and approaches to diagnosis and treatment. Both public and private funds for development were readily available in the free enterprise atmosphere of the years following the introduction of Medicare.

Increasing utilization of the new technologies was fueled by patient demand and the rising cost of defending against malpractice claims. Defensive medicine became the rule, fueling further increases in health care costs in general and escalating the insurance company response. Because the health care system lacked a means of assessing the efficacy of the new technologies, their use grew unchecked, creating major compensatory dissonances. Prominent among these were the cost, uneven distribution, and unresolved bioethical issues of technology use.

DRGs: The Turning Point

The single most dramatic example of compensatory dissonance occurred with the introduction of DRGs. Having failed to find solutions in concert with elements of the health care system, the federal government embarked on its own war on costs. HCFA's Medicare program, which had been such a boon to providers, now became a weapon: the vast quantities of patient information that hospitals had given to HCFA were used to devise the system of DRGs.

This artificial grouping of diseases for purposes of defining HCFA's payment to the hospital created upheaval in the hospital industry. It necessitated a nontrivial changeover of computer systems and the retraining of personnel. Worse, it changed the very goals and incentives that governed the way hospitals operated. For example, prior to the introduction of DRGs, testing in such ancillary departments as laboratory or X ray generated income for the hospital; with DRGs, the fixed payment per case has meant that the hospital has a financial incentive to conduct fewer tests for Medicare patients. Whereas more tests used to mean more income, now fewer tests conserve income.

For their very survival, hospitals have found several ways to compensate for the effects of the DRG system. However, many of these moves caused further dissonance. Cost shifting to non-Medicare patients has helped feed the rise in insurance premiums; DRG creep has kept costs artificially inflated; shorter hospital stays have contributed to higher rates of nursing home admissions and hospital readmissions; and in their search for additional revenues, most hospitals have embarked on expensive new programs, such as outpatient centers, affiliations with other hospitals in the region, and marketing services to the public.

Meanwhile, the cost spiral was having a profound effect on insurance companies, and premiums have skyrocketed. Many companies hedged against an uncertain future by starting their own managed-care operations. Such changes as increased experience rating, reduced coverage, and the preauthorization requirement have created further compensatory dissonances in the system by contributing to the worsening problem of access. Other third-party payers such as state governments have reacted and contributed similarly to the dissonance by shrinking the pool of people covered by Medicaid and reducing coverage.

The System Today

We have today a complex acute medical care system that is preoccupied with its advanced technology and with maintaining the institutional autonomy of each of its constituent elements—to the point of neglecting the health of the population it is supposed to serve. It is also a prosperous system, the development of which has far outpaced its ability to manage itself. Moreover, it is a system without leadership and in serious danger of losing control over its every function. Each of these characteristics, the evolution of which can be seen in the preceding examples and discussion, are examined more closely below, as a prelude to a prediction of what the future holds.

Advanced Technology

The impact of advanced technology has contributed substantially to the problems of health care access and cost in several different ways. Among these are fostering the proliferation of specialties and specialists and outpacing our ability to evaluate its value to the health of the population.

Although technology users encompass a complex array of quantities and types of providers, such as physicians, nurses, social workers, and technologists, they almost all use the technology at the pleasure of a physician. In fact, the physician community continues to be the pivotal element of the health care system's function. Thus this discussion of advanced technology focuses on its evolutionary impact on the physician community.

The physician community has evolved to become a body of highly trained providers of acute care whose practitioners are collectively quite removed from the concerns of public health and the linkages between health and other social parameters. The physician community is swollen with specialists and is ill equipped to deliver most of the primary care needed in the United States, including preventive care and education. There simply are not enough primary care physicians to deliver all the primary care that is needed. Those we do have did not receive the training they would need while they were in medical school. The overproduction of specialists continues because, although residency programs must be accredited, there is no mechanism within the specialties or within the health care system as a whole to control the number and kinds of specialists trained or their distribution throughout the country.

Further, whether specialists or primary care providers, physicians long ago lost the race to keep up with the dizzying pace of new research and the development of new technology. All too often, important new information takes years to find its way into medical school curricula and into the review articles that many physicians rely on. Moreover, the information that does reach physicians can be inadequate for the needs of medical practice.

In their article on the quality of medical evidence, Eddy and Billings (1988, p. 20) argue that "for at least some important practices, the existing evidence is of such poor quality that it is virtually impossible to determine even what effect the practice has on patients, much less whether that effect is preferable to the outcomes that would have occurred with other options. Furthermore, whatever the quality of the existing evidence, our current ability to analyze that information is primitive. As a consequence of these two findings, we simply do not know the appropriate standard of care for some medical practices. The care that is currently being delivered might or might not be appropriate."

Several researchers (Eddy and Billings, 1988; Grimes, 1993; Laffel and Berwick, 1992; Schoenbaum, 1993) have deplored the lack of good evaluation for many extensively used procedures and other technologies. Thus physicians do not have access to good information about expected outcomes. Instead, they must base many important decisions on *belief* rather than *knowledge*. The health care system simply does not have mechanisms whereby new technologies can be routinely evaluated and the results made readily available to practicing physicians.

Unfortunately, even if such information were readily available, most physicians today are not equipped to use

it effectively. This is not the fault of the individual physicians. Rather, we must look to the system that produces
physicians: medical schools and specialist training programs. Both still rely on apprenticeship to teach clinical
skills, and neither prepares physicians to be lifelong learn-
ers who can readily incorporate new findings and technologies into their practices.

The picture today, then, is one of a physician community that is on the verge of losing its increasingly tenuous
grasp on its professional capabilities. It also appears to be
a community without a collective voice. For the past forty
years, it has entrusted its evolution into the modern age
to a trade organization, the AMA, thereby abdicating its
responsibility for professional, ethical, moral, and social
leadership with respect to health care.

Prosperity

The for-profit sector is buying into the health care system
at an escalating rate, a sure sign of the anticipated profitability of health care. By October of 1993, health care acqui-
sitions totaling $15.3 billion had already been announced,
more than doubling the $7.2 billion in acquisitions an-
nounced in all of 1992 (Anders, 1993). Here are some
examples.

> In 1993 and 1994, New York Life Insurance Com-
> pany will add 75 managed-care networks to its base
> of 129 networks (Steinmetz, 1993).
>
> In August of 1993, Columbia Hospital Corporation
> took over Galen Health Care for $3.2 billion in

stock, adding Galen's thirteen hospitals to its base of twenty-six hospitals. Then in October of 1993, Columbia acquired HCA-Hospital Corporation of America's ninety-six hospitals for $5.7 billion in stock (Jones, 1993).

If Health Net, an HMO, completes its merger with QualMed, Inc., managers at Health Net could collect $100 million for the stock for which they paid $1.5 million less than two years earlier ("Health Net Execs," 1993).

It seems reasonable to conclude that these expanded for-profit corporations expect health care to continue to be profitable in the coming years.

Leadership

While it could be argued that health care policy is not the responsibility of the health care system, it has until recently been the expectation of the population that it should be. Certainly the health care system *could* have exercised leadership over its own affairs at any time in the past several decades, thus preempting the external agencies that have stepped in to fill the gap, however inadequately. Following are several examples of the system's failure to lead that will continue to have repercussions into the future.

First of all, the system's failure to take responsibility for the spiraling costs of care is the most dramatic demonstration of the consequences of the failure to lead. This is because critically necessary cost containment measures imposed from outside the system have been shown to be the primary cause of compensatory dissonance within the system. Now the door has been opened to outside manipulation of virtually every aspect of the health care system except its very core, the practitioner-patient relationship. Now the physician community feels compelled to use its limited resources to protect this vital core instead of using them to understand what it must do to help build the health care system we need.

A second critical example is the system's failure to address the class of problems relating to proliferation of advanced technology, especially technology assessment, thus inviting nonhealth care system intervention in the practitioner-patient relationship.

The health care system has also failed to take into account the relationship of medical practice to public health (environment, epidemics) and the relationship of both of these to our worsening social problems (substance abuse, domestic abuse, teenage pregnancy, crime, poverty, social alienation). Moreover, the system has failed to take responsibility for wellness and prevention and to provide leadership in coping with the most painful of all bioethical issues, the gray areas of the beginning and end of life.

The physician community in particular has failed to take the lead in regulating itself as a profession by taking responsibility for the number, kind, distribution, training, professionalism, and quality of practice of its members.

Finally, the system has failed to use any but the most rudimentary tools and techniques of systems and management sciences, such as planning, record keeping, and information technology, to keep its complex house in order.

Unfortunately, the system does not have mechanisms whereby it could begin to exercise leadership; neither is any group outside the health care system equipped to take on these tasks. Thus the system is truly out of control in the sense that no one is in control.

If Existing Trends Continue

It seems highly unlikely that any of the evolutionary trends we have been examining will be mitigated soon; if they do continue into the future, the health care system in the year 2000 will be easy to predict. The examples of compensatory dissonance from the past are a template for those of the near future.

Unacceptably high costs will understandably continue to dominate the health care agenda. In response, sheer survival concerns will guide the actions of most stakeholders as they try to function under the mounting pressure to cut costs. As individual stakeholders, they have no real way of cutting or even containing costs because doing so would not be compatible with survival. The system is so complex and the elements are so interlocked that costs can only be contained by cooperative planning and action. However, without a mechanism or even an agreement in principle to do this, cost containment appears impossible in the near term. Instead, what follows is the likely path of each stakeholder's evolution over the next several years, if the system is allowed to continue to evolve as it has in the past.

The Biggest Payer: Government

Because of its enormous annual investment in health care, the federal government is likely to continue giving cost containment its highest health care priority, with improved access a close second. It will assume the lead in creating the next set of dissonances by taking several successive actions toward improved access and cost control. The initial scenarios of government actions and system reactions—tax increases and incentives to use HMOs—are discussed first.

Managed care is generally believed to be the most likely mechanism available with the capability of reducing the cost of delivering health care, and so it figures prominently in the government's plans as a way of extending health care to all Americans. Taxes will finance the new coverage. The belief is that the cost spiral will be damped by greater use of prepaid care throughout the system.

Regardless of the form it takes, the new government spending will give a boost to the economy because new organizations, facilities, and jobs will have to be created. Further, people not now in the health care system will tend to use health care services differently. New kinds of programs that focus on such areas as patient education and follow-up, prevention, and community outreach will be developed.

The government's new program of access for all Americans soon will have established a formal two-tiered system of health care, and many procedures will not be available to those without private insurance. Setting the resulting class action lawsuits against the government will further add to the health care bill.

With so many health care delivery organizations springing up, including many new types of organizations, it will be very difficult to assess the quality and value of all their activities. Consequently, the extent of their impact—good or bad—on quality of care will not be known for several years. Before very many years have passed, however, Americans will find that the new taxes did not begin to pay for the real cost of adding millions of people to the health care system.

In the next round of health care cost cutting, the government will institute price freezes, abolish malpractice suits, and begin extensive regulation of the insurance industry and other for-profit providers of health-related goods and services. In fee-for-service health care, as was the case during the price freeze of the 1970s, *more* procedures will be done and periods of care will be longer so that provider financial expectations can be met. In prepaid health plans, *fewer* procedures will be done so that provider financial expectations can be met. Suppliers of health-related goods, such as pharmaceutical companies, will cut back on research programs, which for years have been diminishingly profitable, and put more funds into public relations and marketing.

Prepaid Managed-Care Providers

Many new HMO-type organizations and many new physicians will be needed. HMOs will compete for physicians by offering financial incentives. New money in health care will attract investors, and most HMOs will be for-profit organizations. Because cost containment pressure will continue unabated and investors always have expectations, HMO physicians will be offered additional incentives to help keep costs down. These physicians will be expected to follow treatment guidelines established by their respective HMOs. In most cases, patients will only see a physician after being screened by a nonphysician. Preventive care and wellness programs will focus on avoiding those medical conditions that are the most expensive to treat.

Newfangled Hospitals

It is fortunate that the hospital industry is resilient because we are already witnessing the breakup of the industry as we know it. The modern tradition of obtaining patients through referral by staff physicians will no longer sustain hospitals. Increasingly, they will use scarce resources to compete with each other and with HMOs and other new types of provider organizations, marketing their programs to organized consumer-representative groups and thus diverting dollars "from patient care to highly paid administrators and proliferating bureaucratic controls" (Andreopoulos, 1993). To survive, many hospitals will forge alliances with other providers to become "integrated health care providers." In all cases, they will offer many new services, including outpatient clinics, community education, and home health care.

Some hospitals and integrated providers will be fortunate enough to compete successfully and make a smooth transition to the new way of doing business. However, many of those that initially fail to win a substantial share of the new health care money will be considered to be second-class providers in their communities. They very likely will not have the resources to compete for subsequent opportunities or to carry out promised new programs. As with HMOs, quality of patient care will be in danger of becoming secondary to organizational imperatives.

Enterprising Insurance Companies

Many insurance companies have already established HMO-type subsidiaries as an alternative to the fee-for-service arrangement, and more will follow. These companies will no longer be able to deny coverage to anyone, and they will routinely offer a wide variety of plans. Their profitability will be protected by the payment they receive for shouldering the burden of coordinating and evaluating the new approaches and organizations. In the second round of government cost cutting, insurance company regulation will be increased to redress the flaws of the first set of changes. All payers will be required to use the same common billing and reporting forms. The changes will be too much for many companies, and a substantial number of carriers will drop out of the health care business.

The Lonely Physician

To maintain an adequate patient base, physicians will increasingly affiliate themselves with one or more provider organizations, each of which will expect a physician to follow its organization-wide guidelines in diagnosing and treating patients. Physicians will feel that their worst fears about "cookbook medicine" are coming true. Paperwork will continue to increase, and fee schedules similar to the RBRVS will become common, further squeezing physicians' income. Patients will be better informed and will put pressure on physicians to become better informed themselves about new developments. Many professionally isolated physicians will feel that medicine is no longer as attractive a profession as it used to be, and some of them will stop practicing to devote full-time to their previously ancillary business enterprises.

The Shift in Research Emphasis

As health care reels from an excess of the fruits of research, medical research will become more focused on specific, well-defined problems such as AIDS, cancer, and primary care. More emphasis will be placed on the sorely needed evaluation of existing technologies as well. Early results will quickly be made widely available, thus contributing to the move toward "cookbook medicine," which many believe is needed to control costs in the managed-care environment.

The Straight Path of Medical Education

Continuing new developments in highly specialized areas such as genetics and microsurgery will lead to even further subspecialization. New physicians will have an even greater detachment from primary care. Public health will fall even farther behind as an educational priority, and epidemics as serious as the AIDS epidemic will become a threat.

On the other hand, the new government funding of care for people who are currently outside the system will increase the demand for primary care providers. Medical schools will again be selectively funded to increase their enrollments to take up the slack. Both public and private institutions will offer incentives to students to select family practice. HMOs and other provider organizations will initiate more internship and residency programs in primary care areas. Medical centers coping with declining patient populations will enter into arrangements with new provider organizations in order to have enough patients to support their training programs and fill their hospital beds.

Alert, Angry Consumers

Television, books, magazines, and newspapers will become sources of extensive health care information for consumers. Better-informed consumers will increasingly pressure their physicians to justify decisions. They will turn more to alternative methods of care as well, and they will demand that these methods be evaluated and included as covered services in their health plans. Consumers who feel they have been victimized by excessive reliance on diagnostic or therapeutic guidelines in their provider organizations will begin to look for relief in the courts.

Matters of Bioethics

Decisions involving the most personal of ethical issues, especially those dealing with medical care at the beginning and end of life, will be made increasingly by third-party payers and HMO administrations.

The Lesson of the Profits

It is hard to imagine that, under the circumstances described above, the health care system at the dawning of the new millennium will be any more desirable than it is now. Quality of care from the patient's point of view is certain to suffer if the kinds of cost containment measures just outlined are at all successful. To those who believe that the foregoing scenarios of what will happen over the next seven or eight years are exaggerated, one could accurately say that we are already on the course. Too many examples exist at the extremes of managed care already. On the one hand, HMOs are believed to offer a very rewarding opportunity to make money ("HMOs Expecting Business to Boom," 1993). On the other hand, when the HMO mechanism is used without due regard for system goals, the compensatory dissonance created can be more than anyone bargained for. Consider the following examples.

Based on the results of the 1992 audit, California state auditors suspended a Medi-Cal (California's Medicaid) contractor from enrolling new clients. At the time of the suspension, the contractor was providing basic outpatient care to fifty-two thousand Medi-Cal clients and in 1992 had won state authorization to enroll up to four hundred thousand new clients despite problems with its 1990 and 1991 audits. The reasons given for the suspension were that the company "delivers substandard medical care, fails to pay its druggist bills on time, and keeps incomplete records" (Robitaille, 1993). The state had earlier received protests about the company's aggressive marketing tactics as well.

Humana found that its health plan (insurance) and hospital businesses were incompatible after it became an integrated health care provider in the early 1980s. Problems developed on the hospital side when the health plan side tried to cut hospital usage and costs. In early 1993, Humana split into two publicly traded companies, effectively separating its insurance and hospital interests (Schiller, 1993).

These examples are harbingers of what can be expected if cost cutting continues on its collision course with patient care. California's fruitless search for cost-effective care and Humana's expensive experiment are likely to be repeated many times over the next ten years, to the extent that profit taking will further stress the system.

The Option to Change

It must be remembered that the rather unpleasant scenarios that opened the preceding section portray what will happen *only if the system continues to act and react in the same manner as it has for the past forty years.* The health care system has the option to change its direction, but only if it is willing first to come to an understanding of the fundamental nature of the problems to be solved. Then it can design the health care system of the future and plan how to achieve it.

As an example, consider one of the important factors thought to be contributing heavily to the cost spiral: the aging of the population. Aging of the population is not a "problem" one can "solve." What we *can* do, however, is anticipate this demographic trend and plan in advance for our response as a society and as a health care system. Health care costs are not rising because the population is aging; they are rising because the health care system is responding inappropriately to the health care needs of an aging population. For instance, the focus for the elderly should perhaps be on better health education, better preventive care, and affordable home care, temporary nursing home care, and hospice care rather than on the use of extensive medical technology.

Another example deals with the problem of achieving better access to health care. The system could take the responsibility of anticipating and planning for the number and kind of specialists needed, especially relative to the number of primary care physicians needed. It could even plan on ways to ensure that people in underserved areas such as the inner city have adequate health resources.

Thus, high costs and unacceptably limited access to care are *symptoms* of underlying processes that must be changed before the symptoms can be effectively relieved. Pouring more money into the system or changing the way the money is channeled to providers will not impact the underlying problems because those at whom these "solutions" are directed—doctors and hospitals—do not have the mechanisms or the power to make the necessary changes. When we assume that they *can* make significant changes, we are trivializing the magnitude of the problem. A key part of the process of achieving the system we want will be to empower the correct change agents.

A Summary of the Issues

The layers of our health care system, like those of an onion, have been clearly shown.

- On the outside are the layers of a state-of-the-art system suffering from out-of-control costs and less than acceptable access to health care.

- Just below the surface and somewhat less apparent are the incipient crises in quality of care, public health, and bioethics.

- Next come the well-studied reasons for the system's flaws: overuse of technology, administrative and bureaucratic waste, overspecialization, maldistribution of physicians, and the threat of malpractice payments.

- Hidden inside these reasons are such less visible causes as private sector profit taking, anachronistic management, failure to set goals for health care, inappropriate medical education, failure to deal with critical bioethical issues, and the general ignorance of almost everyone from policy makers to consumers about what it is that doctors do or should do.

- At the core of the system are the forces on which it has been built: the unmanaged explosion of knowledge and information, the lack of infrastructure, and the failure of leadership.

As a society we cannot stop at the first few layers as we look for solutions to the problems in the system. Now that the core has been exposed, our efforts must take into account what has been revealed there.

Chapter Four

Nine Critical Questions

Given what we know about key characteristics and under-lying forces in health care, we can now consider the ex-tent to which the present system can or cannot respond to current and future manifestations of crisis. Focusing on the cost and access issues, this chapter poses a series of questions designed to show how the current system is un-able to respond effectively to demands that it either change or compensate for the perceived causal factors. We shall see that while individual institutions or groups can address each of the problems without systemwide cooperation, there are limits to what each group can do alone.

Why Are Cost-Reducing Pressures on Doctors and Hospitals Unrealistic?

Excessive costs in the system are generally thought to be due to wasteful administrative practices, overuse of tech-nology, and excess profit taking by health care–related businesses. Let's take a closer look at how the system deals with each of these issues.

Administrative Waste

Individual health care institutions, especially hospitals and prepaid groups but not most outpatient facilities, have tightened their operations and experienced significant cost savings over the past decade. They have done this by introducing information technology and management techniques, such as performance monitoring and quality improvement, that have been used successfully in other industries. Most continue to make further improvements at the margins, but there are limits to what they can do as individual institutions. The trend toward multi-institutional corporations should facilitate further economies of scale through the use of common record systems and cost and service tracking, but there are still limits.

The era of accountability we are entering will further exacerbate administrative costs for both individual institutions and groups of institutions. The next step needs to be systemwide progress toward reducing duplication of effort among institutions on a national basis. Consider the following examples.

Uniform cost accounting and pressures for accountability in several arenas on a national level will increase provider groups' costs unless and until those providing and seeking information agree on standard requirements, record systems, and communications systems. Currently, provider groups are each developing their own—mostly incompatible—approaches, which will prove costly to make compatible later. But the health care system does not have a mechanism whereby all stakeholders can work together now to make plans for cost containment on a national level.

When patients move, change doctors, or see a consultant, repetitive history taking, examinations, and testing are common. Information technology makes this waste of resources unnecessary, but only if provider groups can agree on a systemwide commitment to common medical record systems, electronic access to remote information, and high-quality testing and data collection. The last of these would require changes in the certification of facilities and the education of health professionals.

Although the waste of resources is a solvable problem, the health care system does not have the infrastructural elements needed to define, plan for, and solve it. In the emerging health care climate, institutions, groups, associations, and agencies appear to be moving toward a competitive rather than a cooperative working relationship—a practice the system cannot afford. Until provider groups work cooperatively on systemwide problems such as the foregoing, the cost of replicating developments across all providers will more than replace whatever institutional savings might have been achieved otherwise.

Overuse of Technology

Technology refers to all medical processes and procedures, including testing, monitoring, and treatments such as drugs and surgery. Some of the reasons for the costly overuse of technology, or overtech, among well-intentioned physicians are given here.

> Even before a new technology has been thoroughly evaluated, physicians may decide to use it on the basis of anecdotal or informal evidence.

Physicians may not be aware of information that would mitigate against the use of a technology. For example, new research findings about alternative approaches may take years to become widely available in books, reviews, and other learning materials.

Physicians may receive new information such as results of a new study and act on the new information because they do not have the time or skills to integrate the new information with existing practices.

Physicians may have a philosophical bias against simpler, alternative therapies, such as chiropractic instead of drugs or surgery.

Physicians may not know how to deliver simpler, less costly therapies such as dietary counseling.

Physicians may fail to use available information. This occurs, for instance, when physicians fail to create and/or follow a sound plan for differential diagnosis and treatment and when they fail to use outcome information compiled from their own collective practice records to guide them in further diagnosis and treatment planning.

Physicians may practice systematic and intentional overtech to counteract potential malpractice claims.

Overtech occurs in the absence of incentives to use technology judiciously.

For all but the last reason, cutting payments to providers will not materially affect the problem of overtech. Clinicians need far better, integrated, and more timely information than they now have to assist them in clinical decision making. Guidelines for the appropriate use of technology should be developed and enforced by the professional community on a national basis, but efforts in that direction are just beginning.

The development of new technology has far outpaced the ability of the system to study its efficacy adequately, although this need not be the case. Today, even when physicians have general information about the efficacy of a particular group of technologies, the information may still not help them very much in making a decision about a particular patient. A corollary to not having needed information about specific efficacy is that physicians must of necessity act on the information that they do have and believe, no matter how fragmentary or out of date it is.

Even when the information a physician needs exists, the health care system does not have an effective mechanism of getting that information to the individual physician. Nor do most physicians have the necessary education, training, or orientation to obtain and integrate new information routinely into their practices.

Systematic overtech to avoid malpractice claims is possible to the extent that it is today because in many cases there are few guidelines as to what tests and treatments would be considered appropriate. (See the discussion of clinical guidelines in the next major section of this chapter.) Overutilization can thus only really be detected after the fact. If guidelines were widely available and accepted, most malpractice cases could be avoided in the first place or quickly settled by reference to these guidelines.

It may seem that guidelines should be unnecessary because the purpose of physician education is to learn what acceptable medical practice is. In fact, there is so much medical information that a physician cannot learn and retain it all. Further, the physician's medical knowledge must be continuously updated. Systemwide changes beyond the scope of individual providers or groups must therefore precede effective control of costs due to the overuse of technology.

Profit Taking

The magnitude of profit taking in health care is not well studied. Physician practices, private hospitals, integrated provider organizations, ancillary medical services such as laboratories and radiology centers, HMOs, insurance companies, drug companies, and other suppliers and contractors to the health care system all profit from health care. This diversity alone makes it almost impossible to get a true picture of the impact of profit taking in health care. Additionally, most of these entities are not publicly owned, making information very difficult to obtain.

Per se, profiting from health care enterprises is not objectionable. When a system is as financially stressed as the health care system is, however, it seems likely that profit taking will be raised as an ethical issue. In any case, it is beyond the scope of individual providers to reconcile profit taking and the conservation of national resources.

Why Must Quality Be Sacrificed to Achieve Lower Costs?

Until the early 1980s, cost was a secondary concern in the health care system. For decades, the trend had been to produce more research, build more hospitals, graduate more and smarter doctors, create more specialties, offer more and better therapies, and appropriate more money to care for more people. Now, opportunities abound for cost saving at the national level, but the system is powerless to act. The system simply does not have any mechanisms for self-examination or self-evaluation to determine the need for or the direction of cost cutting. Nor does it have the ability to implement cost cutting or any other major change, no matter how worthy. The system has no power to close hospitals, lower medical school enrollments, or terminate residency programs except for cause, to redirect research and development, or to prevent providers from indiscriminate use of new developments.

In the absence of a systemwide response to cost-cutting pressures, the pressures fall primarily on provider groups, which are also powerless to act in these areas. As noted earlier, most providers have gone about as far as possible in cutting costs in administrative—nonmedical—areas; incentives are powerful to make services the next intra-provider target. As we have seen from the discussion of overtech, providers cannot really impact clinical decision making except through administrative guidelines for productivity, quotas, rationing, use of gatekeepers, selective use of preventive medicine, and reliance on institutional quality indicators. From the patient's point of view, these are hardly quality-oriented actions.

Why Aren't Clinical Guidelines Available?

Because overtech is thought to be a significant contributor to excessive costs, one approach to containment that is gaining support is to give physicians better guidance in clinical decision making. Increasingly, physicians are having to accept the involvement of outsiders in clinical decisions. Insurance companies and hospitals look over physicians' shoulders, and government agencies and professional groups such as specialty societies offer guidelines. The question is no longer whether physicians will accept such guidance but whether such guidance, as it is available today, has any practical value.

Guideline development uses a blend of such resources as literature review, expert opinion and consensus, and directed research. Standards for developing and testing guidelines are just beginning to emerge; the problems of dissemination, use, and updating lie ahead (Owens and Nease, 1993). The relatively new field of outcomes research is the area of interest.

Outcomes research studies the efficacy and safety of procedures (tests, treatments, and other processes) used in health care. A typical research study focuses on a specific population with a specific problem; it compares specific procedures and attempts to draw conclusions about the best way to approach the problem. All forms of good research that use today's tools and techniques are exacting, expensive, and time-consuming, and the problem of integrating new, specific findings with already existing knowledge is formidable. Because research is too broad a subject to be considered extensively in this book, only a few ideas are discussed to illustrate the difficulties.

Typically, outcomes research follows one of three schemes, each of which has its drawbacks: (1) prospective studies, in which studies are planned in advance of data collection (including clinical trials); (2) retrospective studies, in which data already existing in medical records and collected for some other purpose are used; or (3) meta-analyses, in which a study is made of several other studies whose results are combined.

Prospective Studies

When a new test or device needs to be approved, prospective research in the form of clinical trials is almost always conducted. Clinical trials are the most exacting form of outcomes research, and they are often carried out at more than one institution by health professionals who are not trained in research. Because clinical trials are so difficult to do well, fairly narrow research questions are asked; as a result, the findings may not be widely applicable. Further, clinical trials usually only compare a new drug or device to a standard one; they do not comment on the value or cost-effectiveness of the new one. Finally, as they are performed today, clinical trials only describe what happened to a typical group of people; they do not predict what will happen to a specific individual patient who will receive the test or treatment in the future.

Genentech's latest study comparing its clot-busting drug, tissue plasminogen activator (TPA), to streptokinase offers an example of several of these points (Petit, 1993). Genentech undertook the study after it concluded that two earlier studies were flawed and the results were inconclusive. The new multiyear study was conducted at a cost of $55 million; it involved forty-one thousand patients in sixteen nations and 1,050 hospital emergency rooms. The findings revealed that one additional life would be saved per hundred heart attack victims treated. The incremental cost of treating one hundred people with TPA instead of streptokinase to save that life would be $180,000. Ironically, according to Dr. Ralph Brindis, who is quoted by Petit, "The key is not what drug or treatment you get, but that you get treatment quickly." Nonetheless, Genentech pronounced the study, which they paid for, a great success.

Prospective studies can also be conducted by following into the future the medical course of groups of people who are selected or categorized according to specific characteristics (cohorts). For example, in 1986 Giovannucci and others (1993a) began a cohort study of approximately fifty thousand male health professionals, about ten thousand of whom had had vasectomies. Using initial and follow-up questionnaires as well as medical records and pathology reports to confirm prostate cancer diagnoses over the ensuing four years, the study concluded that vasectomy increases the risk of prostate cancer.

This kind of study is also expensive, time-consuming, and difficult to do well, so it is typically very limited in scope. For instance, although this study used health professionals, who presumably are more knowledgeable than the average patient, self-reporting of diagnoses, test results, treatments, or even symptoms is not a very reliable way to gather data. Even when a study such as this one is well conducted, it may not offer much guidance to physicians and patients in individual situations where the risk of prostate cancer must be weighed against the value and side effects of a vasectomy.

Retrospective Studies

Retrospective studies examine events that have already occurred. In contrast to the preceding study, consider a retrospective study on vasectomy and prostate cancer, also conducted by Giovannucci and others (1993b). Questionnaires were used to determine whether or not about twenty thousand nurses' husbands—half of whom had been determined by questionnaire in 1972 to have had vasectomies—had developed prostate cancer in the intervening years. Following verification, the retrospective study also concluded that vasectomy increases the risk of prostate cancer.

Retrospective studies usually rely on data already collected primarily from medical records. However, medical records are simply not designed to be research tools, and they are not treated as such when they are created. Quality is a serious problem. Access to medical records and the information they contain is also a serious problem. There is no external index that gives clues to which records might be useful for a study. A record itself is difficult to review, even by the people who created it.

Meta-Analysis

Meta-analysis is a promising study technique that has the potential to offer more powerful conclusions by combining the results of several related studies conducted in the past. To be unbiased, however, meta-analysis requires that *all* appropriate related studies be used, so both national and international literature must be searched exhaustively. Once retrieved, further analysis typically shows that far too many of the original studies were flawed and are not usable. Some of the earlier studies relied on designs, populations, or other factors that make them inappropriate for combination. Unfortunately, it is not possible to use meta-analysis in many important cases where the disease or procedure in question had been thought to have been well studied.

Criteria for New Types of Research

The discussion has pointed to the inadequacy of current research techniques as a major factor preventing the health care system from assessing adequately the efficacy of its portfolio. These techniques are most useful when the disease process is well defined and follows about the same course in everyone who contracts it and when the outcome measure is easily identified. But most of the "easy" studies have already been done.

One problem plaguing outcomes research is defining meaningful outcomes to measure (Siu and others, 1992). While Siu's concern is for the impact of improved care on health, current measures range all the way from the mortality rate for certain procedures in hospitals to cost of care to patient satisfaction!

Assessing a patient's potential for good quality of life and subjective opinions about the desirability of procedures have become increasingly important. For instance, at one time it was important just to survive breast cancer; today additional treatment options have made it possible to consider survival without extensive disfigurement. Yet disfigurement is still preferred by those who fear radiation or do not trust chemical treatments—regardless of the relative efficacy. Thus, outcomes research aimed at producing guidance for physicians would need to take into account many more, often subjective, factors than it does now.

Much of the confusion about the relative efficacy of different technologies today seems to stem from the fact that different things "work" for different people and a "successful" or "best" outcome is not always well defined. For instance, it seems likely that there are breast cancer patients for whom mastectomy is clearly the better choice and other breast cancer patients for whom radiation is clearly the better choice. Often, however, we don't know which patients are which. The same is true for medical versus surgical treatment of atherosclerotic heart disease and for knee surgery options. Many valuable research resources have been wasted because of our inability to define target populations adequately. For guidelines to have any value, research techniques need to be directed toward defining correct target populations.

Drug research is another example of where better defined target populations are needed. When technologies such as new drug therapies are applicable to smaller and smaller subsets of the population, it is increasingly difficult to find enough people with the necessary problems for inclusion in traditional kinds of studies. As a result, the cost of new drug research, in terms of time and resources, can be expected to continue to rise.

Medical Records as a Research Tool

Medical records, as noted above, could be an invaluable source of research information. For instance, if medical records had been routinely harvested by researchers, the shocking geographical practice variations and the extensive unnecessary use of technology could have been detected and mitigated years before they became serious contributors to the cost spiral (Wennberg, Freeman, and Culp, 1987). Medical records could also be used routinely to identify characteristics of likely target populations for treatment alternatives. However, medical records are not treated as dynamic documents that contain vital clues to the course of diseases under a wide variety of situations. The quality and accessibility of information in medical records is less than adequate, so they cannot today be considered as essential tools of research, education, and consultation.

Dissemination of Research Findings

Several questions should be asked about the dissemination of research findings. Does the research have sufficient validity and value to the physician that it should be disseminated? How are the findings physically disseminated? Does the physician have the ability to integrate the new information into her or his existing base of knowledge and to use it in practice? Each of these questions is considered below.

Value of research. We have already touched on the inadequacy of much research for solving the contemporary physician's daily dilemmas because of its limited scope. Further, direct interpretation of studies is beyond the ability of most physicians, who generally receive little training in such research concepts as probability theory or statistical inference. Study findings therefore need to be interpreted and put in context by experts prior to dissemination.

Physical dissemination. Existing mechanisms such as conferences, review articles, and continuing medical education opportunities have failed to meet the need for physical dissemination of information to physicians. Electronic indexes and abstracts are available through the National Library of Medicine's MEDLINE, but they are laborious to use and not widely accepted by practicing physicians. For those who can and do access information electronically, the information, again, is almost always available only in a form that is without reference to the context of the physician's need for it.

Integration into practice. The context of a physician's need is the critical element in determining the usefulness of disseminating information. The physician needs to be able to ask specific questions about a case at hand and receive specific guidance that incorporates a synthesis of all relevant factors. Alternatively, new information could be incorporated into guidelines of sufficient scope to cover most clinical situations.

In summary, then, outcomes research as it is presently conducted is expensive and time-consuming. The invaluable resources of good past studies and high-quality, accessible medical records are not generally available. For most of medical practice, there is no coordinated plan to set standards and define guidelines. The health care system is investing relatively few resources in investigating issues related to dissemination. Finally, changes in medical education that would help the physician cope with emerging payer and patient expectations are not on the horizon.

Why Are New Technologies Extensively Used Before They Are Thoroughly Evaluated?

For new drugs or devices to be approved by the Food and Drug Administration (FDA), they need only be found to be reasonably safe and effective. Other new processes and procedures such as laboratory tests and surgical procedures are not required to have any validation at all; they can be introduced and used simply on the basis of belief in their value. Thus new technologies may be used for years on thousands of patients before tests are conducted to compare them to other options or before countervailing factors are known and acted on. Even today, only costly procedures are being evaluated extensively.

Because effective evaluation can be very difficult and because it has not often been required, it has not often been done. Except for the limited interests of the FDA and the limited activities of certain professional associations, the health care system does not have an infrastructural mechanism for assessment of old or new technologies.

Why Isn't There More Emphasis on Preventive Care and Wellness?

People need and expect the health care system to deliver health education and preventive care and to provide all necessary facilities and services to care for their health problems. Ironically, most people are unaware of the fact that this is not what they are getting. Consumers are generally unaware of the extent to which their lives could be healthier, safer, and more comfortable if the health care system pursued the goals of better preventive care and wellness.

At the level of the individual physician-patient relationship, the patient is shortchanged. Our family physicians had to learn so much "medicine" that they did not have time to learn how to practice holistic health care or how to keep their patients healthy. Further, most were not taught to use the management skills and tools that would enable them to schedule effectively the essential routine testing and other procedures of prevention and early detection. For instance, if a patient does not remember to schedule a mammogram or immunization or ignores or forgets a reminder, the busy physician's office is not likely to notice and the procedure will not be done. Community outreach, to ensure that such follow-up and other routine education and care are given, is outside the conceptual framework of both individual providers and the health care system.

The health care system and virtually every element within it are geared toward caring for and curing the acutely ill patient. The providers of care—primarily physicians and hospitals—are equipped to deliver acute care; health care personnel are taught acute care; the payment system pays for acute care. There are no mechanisms—organizational structure, institution, financing method, including managed care, or personnel—whose responsibility it is to help people stay healthy, avoid illnesses, or manage chronic problems.

Nor is the health care system well integrated with the larger social system of which it is a part. Systems theory tells us that a sound health care system would need to respect and work toward the goals of society. But the system does not take into account an extensive array of critical social factors that impinge on the health of individuals and affect their use of the health care system. These factors include substance abuse, teen pregnancy, violence, poverty, illiteracy, environmental effects, and industrial and other accidents. Although many people consider these to be major causal factors in the use of health care services, they are not thought to be the responsibility of the health care system.

The health care system is so far removed from the social factors of disease that it is even redefining *preventive care*. This term used to mean care to prevent one from getting sick; increasingly, it refers to early detection, not prevention, of disease. For many health care problems, preventive care and subsequent services to the entire population at risk would cost more than treating the problems as they arise. Giving regular mammograms to all women between forty and fifty is a case in point. Thus contemporary preventive care, even in managed-care environments, is directed primarily toward avoiding costly care at the advanced stage of disease rather than trying to prevent it altogether (Barnum, 1993).

The health care system turned its back on public health as an area of concern many years ago. Foege (1992) points to three ways in which preventive medicine and public health are not fulfilling their potential in society. First, old problems such as low levels of immunization, the threat of tuberculosis, and bacterial drug resistance are recurring.

Second, the gaps continue among demographic groups on such measures as infant mortality. Third, scientific knowledge fails to influence public policy adequately in, for instance, the areas of tobacco and alcohol use and caring for children. The tragedy in the United States is that we have the knowledge but do not use it. Foege concludes by saying, "For many Americans there is no advantage to living in a country with such a great public health tradition" (p. 402).

The idea that individuals should take responsibility for their own health is gaining support. However, the knowledge they would need to do so—knowledge about medicine and health—is even more inaccessible to the public than it is to practicing physicians. People need a systematic, reliable, and comprehensive source of guidance and reference information. The medical literature is available, but it is both arcane and physically difficult to access. Magazine and newspaper articles do offer easily understood summary information and updates about specific diseases and technologies, but the information is not very useful in promoting self-responsibility. Medical books and health guides for laypeople are superficial and not very authoritative. Indeed, it would be difficult, given the state of health knowledge today, to offer an adequate resource because, as a discipline, research on health is still in its infancy.

In summary, it could be said that most of the health-related assistance people really need is not being delivered by our acute-care system. This includes systematic provision for consumer health education, wellness programs, prenatal care, care for school-age children, self-care, follow-up care, care for chronic problems, and custodial care for the preservation of health. The system as it exists today has few mechanisms for delivering these kinds of care, except on an exception basis in specific projects and for those who specifically seek it out and can pay for it. Achieving the necessary levels of nonacute care would require a major refocusing of the health care system and a shifting of resources toward maintaining wellness.

Why Is Access to Care Unavailable to So Many People?

The cost of health care is the primary reason for decreasing access to care. Free services have been cut throughout the system; many people who were able to get care in the past, even when unemployed or uninsured, can no longer do so. However, cost is only part of the problem. Demographics also play a role. Access is a pervasive problem in the inner cities and in rural areas almost regardless of the cost of care. The health care system is lacking in incentives to providers to locate in these areas in adequate numbers. It is unrealistic to expect hospitals and clinics to locate in areas where revenues cannot support them. As for physicians, when they are ready to make a decision about the kind of practice in which they will spend their professional lives, they have just finished over ten years of learning at great expense to solve complex medical problems. It is unrealistic to expect them to want to deliver nutrition counseling and well-baby care in low-income areas.

Thus the issue of access goes to the heart of what the

health care system believes its business to be. This is evidenced at least in part by the education and orientation the system gives its practitioners and providers. It does not produce a type of professional whose business it is to understand the totality of the forces and needs in the health care system and who could plan to accommodate and achieve them. Even health policy specialists today are concerned almost exclusively with payment mechanisms and the organization of health care rather than with solving or mitigating the underlying problems of limited access and excessive costs.

Why Don't Medical Schools Prepare Graduates for the Country's Needs?

Medical education today is the product of the information explosion that has occurred over the past several decades and of the laudable desire for medicine to become more and more a modern science. Medical school faculty members are of necessity researchers who are attuned to new ideas and technologies. Their livelihood and the success of their institutions depend on research funding. As there is more and more to know about medicine, there is less and less time in the curriculum to integrate it into the context—which is the human need—of the *practice* of medicine.

Compounding these factors is the archaic method of teaching clinical medicine that has evolved. Clinical medicine is still taught primarily by the apprenticeship method. Students, interns, and residents learn primarily from practicing on the individual patients who happen to be present during their tenure in a clinic. Naturally, the most desirable patients are those with the most interesting medical problems. Further, as more and more patients are turning to prepaid practice plans, medical schools are facing a shortage of primary care patients on whom to practice, at the very time when more primary care physicians are needed.

It is ironic that the medical profession, in its quest to become more of a science and to take full advantage of modern medical technologies, has rushed past computing and communications—the very technologies that could help it cope with exploding medical knowledge. Instead of managing patient information along with accessing medical knowledge as it is needed, most physicians rely primarily on information they remember and believe to be correct. This is what they were taught to do.

The medical education system has evolved so far in the direction of imparting specific medical knowledge that it is now probably impossible to redefine the physician as needing to memorize less of it. This is particularly true of specialists, but it is also true for primary care physicians. Although we may want to add to the list of things our primary care physicians need to understand, no one would care to make a list of the diseases and therapies they no longer need to know about.

Incentives to change the system of medical education are few. The Association of American Medical Colleges and the Council on Graduate Medical Education make recommendations, but changes are voluntary. Some schools experiment periodically with new ways of doing business, but since modern medical education was defined by the

Flexner Report in 1910, the only real systemwide change has been to lengthen the time it takes to become a physician.

Until medical education finds a way to convert its curriculum to one that teaches physicians lifelong learning and information management skills, today's model of an educated physician is unlikely to change. Since there is no policy-making or policy-enforcing body in medical education, any possible change will be voluntary and probably piecemeal. Unfortunately, even if a medical school wanted to make this kind of change, so that there would be more time in the curriculum for teaching the *practice* of medicine, patient information and medical knowledge are not organized in such a way as to make this possible. In the short term it will be necessary to create new models for teaching the delivery of primary care.

What Is the Role of Professional Organizations?

Health professional organizations are primarily either scientific and educational associations or trade associations. The former are concerned with such scholarly aspects of the profession as education; maintenance of members' skills through publications, courses, and conferences; and the processes of certification and accreditation. Physicians are not required to belong to such organizations, and indeed there is no particular scientific or educational association to which most physicians belong. Even the specialty associations do not have the authority to dictate member activities or regulate the number of new graduates in their specialties or where they will practice.

89

The mission of trade associations is to further the interests of their voluntary individual or institutional members. The health industry trade associations are a powerful political force. In addition to spending money for lobbying activities, their political action committees collectively contributed $14.4 million to congressional candidates in 1992. Of that amount, the AMA alone, which represents somewhat less than half of United States physicians, contributed $2.9 million.

Accrediting associations do offer some potential for systemwide action on health care issues. For instance, the Joint Commission on Accreditation of Healthcare Organizations (JCAHO) is using accreditation as the stick to make it mandatory for hospitals to contribute performance indicators to a national database. This move would allow patients and other stakeholders to rate individual providers on the basis of patient outcomes (Skolnick, 1993).

Most health professional organizations are very concerned about health policy, and they issue policy statements ranging from the self-serving to the thoughtful and concerned. However, because almost none of these groups is able to require its members to support or follow specific policies, it cannot be said that there are policy-making groups among the health professional organizations.

Collectively, there is no recognized and widely supported overarching health professional group or collection of groups whose responsibility it is to

- Articulate health care goals for the country
- Make plans for meeting those goals

- Coordinate implementation among all stakeholders
- Assess progress and make needed modifications

Thus there is no group that can say authoritatively and convincingly what it is that physicians should know, what services they should deliver, how they should conduct their practices, what number and kind of physicians are needed, and where they should practice.

Why Does the System Seem So Detached?

The information explosion and the American tradition of private enterprise have run headlong into the awakening American consciousness that health care could be something everyone should have. Added to that is the hard-won professional respect accorded to physicians to the extent that nonmedical people, including health policy makers and most of the general population, do not really know what it is that physicians and the rest of the health care system do or should do. The result is the system we have, which is characterized as being out of balance, expensive, and too inaccessible.

Consideration of these matters collectively sheds light on several key concept-level barriers that are contributing to the health care system's inability to respond appropriately.

- The system has evolved in the absence of an understanding of what the national goals for health care might be.

- The health care system does not really see itself as

a system or organize itself as a system. It appears on close examination to be principally a collection of special interests and altruistic but entrepreneurial organizations reacting to each other but not interacting constructively.

- Health policy makers in general do not appear to realize the complexity of the health care system or the implications of that complexity. They tend to define the system in terms of selected components that they think they understand, such as payment mechanisms, instead of looking for a deeper understanding.

- The system does not have an adequate and constructive relationship with the sociopolitical system of which it is a part or with other elements of the larger system.

- The system has almost reached the end of its ability to continue to evolve. It appears to have reached a state of increasing compensatory dissonance characterized by reflexive response to internal and external stimuli.

- The system has advanced the cause of many of its elements through the use of modern technology; many lives have been saved and the quality of life enhanced for many others. However, the system has failed to use modern information technology to organize and manage itself successfully and to guide the appropriate use of medical technologies.

This analysis of why the health care system cannot respond to its serious crises completes the evidence pointing to the areas of infrastructure, leadership, and information flow as the culprits. It must be well noted that, despite the apparent failure of the health care system as a whole to position itself for continuity into the future, little blame can be attached to individual providers and provider institutions who are delivering the best health care they know how to deliver under less than optimal circumstances.

PART TWO

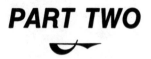

The Power of a New
Health Information System

Chapter Five

The Information Logjam

Inadequate information flow, or an information logjam, occurs when information that exists or should exist in the health care system and outside it is not available for optimal use or is not being used optimally by the system. The answers to the questions in Chapter Four show just how extensively blocked information flow figures as a major underlying problem factor. In most cases the needed information exists; it simply is inaccessible.

In this chapter we narrow in on the information logjam to see how it cuts across the system, preventing solution of current crises and perpetuating them into the future. Let's first define some of the concepts of health information flow and then pinpoint various health areas where information is blocked, in a way that identifies the commonality of the problem throughout the system.

Information Flow Concepts

The following definitions provide a common terminology and an explanation of specific concepts that will be used to discuss information flow and the information logjam.

Medical knowledge is the body of facts on which the practice of health care is based. It is considered to be a relatively fixed body of knowledge that is growing and undergoing constant updating and refinement. Examples of medical knowledge extend to human anatomy and physiology, biochemistry and microbiology, cardiology and endocrinology, the results of medical research, and experience with medical procedures.

Patient information, on the other hand, is highly variable. The patient record is just as meaningful and important as medical knowledge, but its content varies from patient to patient and, for any patient, over time.

Accessibility of information (especially medical knowledge and patient information) involves three requirements: (1) the information must be in a usable form, (2) one must be able to get to it physically, and (3) one must be able to integrate it for optimal use once it is received. Information that exits in memory or in notes, is in a book miles from where it is needed, or is formatted in such a way that it takes a long time to decipher (perhaps as in a research article) would not be considered accessible.

Education as an information flow concept refers both to the education health professionals need so that they can work with information effectively and to the use of information for the process of education.

Research as an information flow concept means both the research needed for better information flow and the need for information flow in research.

Infrastructure as an information flow concept refers to the need for an infrastructure for information flow and also to the need for information flow so that the infrastructure of health care can function properly.

The Medical Knowledge Logjam

The extensive body of medical literature is far beyond the capabilities of most physicians to review routinely. Review articles about specific medical conditions or therapies, which many physicians rely on to stay current, often do not reflect the latest knowledge; sometimes, in fact, they are several years out of date. Recent attempts to make extensive use of meta-analysis have shown that the state of medical knowledge is not as advanced as was previously believed. Definitive studies that could offer genuinely useful guidance to physicians are rare. Thus much more than we would like of the basis for specific medical practices exists in forms that are not very useful (such as in the memories and experiences of specific practitioners) and cannot be readily codified.

The implications of this situation are grave in terms of the overuse and inappropriate use of medical technology, which collectively we have called overtech. Too often, reliable information not only about new technologies but also about many technologies that have been in standard use for years has been unavailable. Coronary artery bypass surgery, endartrectomy, cesarean section, and prostate surgery are recent examples.

Physicians and other caregivers who do not have specific, reliable information about the efficacy and appropriate use of tests, devices, and procedures old and new must rely too much on information from manufacturers, textbooks that may be out-of-date even before publication, their own beliefs, anecdotal evidence, news stories, patient preferences, and possibly inappropriate research articles. Moreover, physicians may not have acquired the research skills needed to detect flawed studies, and other studies may be so narrow in scope that their findings are not applicable to the particular patient a physician wants to help. Still, this may be the best information the physician has.

Physicians are not the only professionals for whom the medical knowledge logjam is a serious problem. As we shall see, nurses, educators, students, researchers, consumers, planners, managers, policy makers, and third-party payers also need accurate and up-to-date medical knowledge.

The Patient Record Logjam

This section considers the consequences of the information logjam for both individual and aggregated patient records.

Individual Records

Although the primary function of the patient record is to assist caregivers with the care of individual patients, the records today do not serve that function very well. As health care has become increasingly complex, the patient record has also grown in size and complexity, but its design has not evolved to keep pace. Following, from a patient care point of view, are some of the primary design flaws that can seriously affect quality of care.

Time integration. Information in the patient record is usually not integrated across time. It is difficult to follow the course of several variables, such as patient parameters or test results, at the same time. Correlation among variables over time is even more difficult to follow.

Section integration. Information elements in the record are not usually correlated with each other. For instance, because laboratory test results are in a different section from nurses' notes or pharmacy records, they can be compared only laboriously.

Comparability. It is difficult for physicians or other caregivers to compare the case at hand with previous similar cases, even at the same institution. Such comparisons could give physicians insights and information that might be useful in making decisions about tests or therapies for the patient. Unless they are willing to make a substantial investment in research or keeping detailed notes, physicians must rely on their memory of the course of other similar medical problems.

Completeness. The patient record exists for the use of the institution that collects the information. The information cannot be correlated readily with the patient's other institutional experiences, with outpatient or home care, or with other highly relevant aspects of the patient's life, such as family or work situation.

Utility. As designed, the information in a patient record cannot be used to benefit the patient to the extent possible. A complete patient record could be routinely analyzed for information that might give insights into problems or potential problems. For example, allergic reactions or contraindicated combinations of medications could be avoided; the patient's progress compared to accepted standards of progress for his or her particular problem could be monitored; adverse events could be flagged; and suggestions could be made for doing and/or avoiding tests or procedures that might not have been considered without extensive analysis of a complete record.

Quality. Record keeping in health care is an ancillary activity. A record that is complete and free of errors will be difficult to achieve unless the health professionals who place information in the record are taught to understand the importance of accuracy and completeness and to give high priority to creating high-quality records.

Aggregated Records

Patient records collectively could be a valuable tool for research, education, consultation, management, and ultimately cost control. However, most of the information they contain is very difficult to use. An information logjam exists because that information is inaccessible for all practical purposes. This particular logjam has had an effect in a number of areas.

Education. Health professional students and residents learn primarily by apprenticeship. This means that they must practice their skills on real patients. Information in patient records, either as cases or groups of cases, could offer a very important educational alternative if it were accessible. To the extent that the system does not make a special effort to make aggregated and individual case histories optimally available as learning tools for students, the students are being shortchanged by an information logjam.

Research. Patient-based research currently requires the laborious, costly, and time-consuming data acquisition that may well not have been necessary if patient records could have been analyzed more readily. The more complete, the higher the quality, and the more accessible patient records are and the easier they are to aggregate, the easier it will be to conduct research. At a minimum, patient records could serve as pointers to questions that cannot be answered from the records alone, and they could help identify target populations so that research could have greater specificity. The limited availability of this information has major implications for clinical research, which in turn affects overtech and cost control.

Consultation. Physicians must rely on their memory of past cases during complex differential diagnosis and treatment planning because they cannot readily review and aggregate information from past patient records. This has implications not only for the quality of individual patient care but also for the ability of physicians to avoid overtech.

Management. Systemwide planners and policy makers have very limited access to patient information except as it has been aggregated for other purposes by institutions and third-party payers. In the absence of complete and reliable information, these individuals must rely on the information they do have, no matter how inappropriate for the problems they are trying to solve. The Health Care Financing Administration's use of billing information to create DRGs and the RBRVS to control costs is a case in point.

As is the case with patient record information used for specific patient care, the *quality* of the information aggregated for use in research, education, and consultation is a major concern. Patient records today have only limited value in research because extensive validation has not been undertaken.

The Accessibility Logjam

The first requirement of accessibility, that the information must exist in a usable form, has not usually been met for either medical knowledge or patient information.

The second requirement, that one must be able to get to the information, is also often unmet. In theory, almost anyone who has access to a medical library, an information service, and/or a computer terminal has access to the medical literature through the National Library of Medicine's MEDLINE. In fact, however, this kind of access is not practical for any group except researchers. Bodies of information that are not as well organized, such as the literature on health and public health or information that could be derived from aggregated patient records, are even less available—to providers as well as educators and students, researchers, consumers, policy makers, and payers.

The third requirement of accessibility is that the information must be relevant and useful in the time, place, and context of the reason for which it is sought. A busy physician simply cannot conduct a computer search, read research publications, and integrate new knowledge with old knowledge and patient information during the course of a day in the hospital or the office. By day's end, priorities have shifted and the moment is lost. Further, the physician often has no way of knowing that there is more information to be had.

To the extent that new knowledge is not integrated in

time, place, and context with information the physician already has, accessibility presents a primary information logjam. This has implications for quality of care and for overtech and cost control, as discussed earlier.

The Education Information Logjam

The health education process contributes to the information logjam because physicians and other health professionals learn very little in school about the invaluable role of information flow in health care. They do not learn to take responsibility for the quality of information they provide to the system, and they do not learn how to access, assess, integrate, and use information as the indispensable resource it could be in their practices. Instead, the learning focus is on memorization and style rather than the development of lifelong learning, case management, and other information-using skills.

At the same time, the educational process is a part of the information logjam when it does not use or make available information tools that could powerfully enrich the learning process. Medical schools collectively could take primary responsibility for research and development of methods and tools for accessing, assessing, and integrating medical knowledge and patient information. Such tools exist in only limited form for use by students, health professionals, patients, and other consumers who want to learn about health and the practice of medicine.

The Information Logjam in Research

While all types of research rely extensively on information flow, an equally important aspect of research is that the health care system has major information gaps—which can only be filled by further research.

Medical Knowledge

Extensive research of all kinds is needed to fill the gaps in the medical knowledge base and to keep it up-to-date. This is particularly important for clinical medicine, where the gaps need to be filled so that quality of care can continue to improve and costs caused by overtech can be contained. Prevention, diagnosis, and treatment of even fairly common diseases such as coronary artery disease are not well understood, and they cannot be well understood using the current approaches to research. For instance, coronary artery disease has many risk factors, but research that uses large numbers of people to satisfy statistical assumptions blurs the subtle differences that would reveal which factors are important for which kinds of people.

Outcomes Research

Although the priority of outcomes research has dramatically improved in recent years, current funding levels afford only the beginning of what needs to be done. A major issue is how to bring societal values and health system goals to bear on definitions of appropriate and acceptable measures of outcomes and standards of practice. Until the health care system formulates and agrees on guidelines and standards, decisions about appropriateness of care will continue to be made by third-party payers, and malpractice allegations will continue to be settled in the court system rather than by professionals.

Pharmaceutical Research

The pharmaceutical industry relies on commercial firms to provide patients for clinical trials and even to manage its research. It also relies extensively on practicing physicians who are not trained in research to administer and monitor new medications. Both of these information-intensive processes would seem to offer scope for improvement in many ways.

Health Services Research

The relatively new and promising field of health services research is limited in the extent to which it can help the health care system learn to manage itself and develop its potential. Because of the difficulty of creating system models for experimentation and analysis, the current focus is on the funding of health care and on micro-organizational issues.

Health Research

For too many Americans, good health still means getting enough vitamins to prevent scurvy or weak bones. If the health education that most physicians give their patients is any indication, that is about all good health means to many physicians as well. Increasingly, health has come to mean more than the absence of illness. Thus research on lifestyle changes and alternative kinds of health care such as chiropractic and acupuncture is becoming recognized as valid. The work is just beginning, however, and much more research is needed.

Random information pertaining to good health is everywhere, but so are the cultural pressures and norms that can lead to unhealthy choices and lifestyles. In the absence of relatively complete, accurate, and authoritative health information that is readily accessible to all consumers, it is unlikely that Americans can be expected to take much responsibility for their own health.

How the Lack of Infrastructure Contributes to the Information Logjam

Without a health care system infrastructure, mechanisms are lacking for the systemwide policy decisions and planning that could make information available on an ongoing basis. Without an infrastructure, information cannot flow throughout the system. As a result, the health care system suffers in at least these ways:

- It has no mechanisms for goal setting and for ensuring that elements of the system understand and work toward set goals.
- It cannot use proven management tools and techniques to deal effectively with such fundamental management issues as providing for access by securing appropriate resources and delivering them to the right places.
- It has not yet understood the benefits of a uniform system of cost accounting.
- It has not yet realized the critical need for, and made a commitment to, supporting outcomes research at the level necessary.

- It has not been able to avoid overtech by developing standards of practice.
- It has not committed adequate resources to the dissemination of knowledge and the flow of information.
- It has not upgraded its educational system in several decades to conform with contemporary health care goals.
- It has little hope of ridding itself of its acute-care orientation, substituting instead a system where acute care is balanced with other components of a healthy life.

Overarching Logjam Issues

Several overarching issues should be evident by now. Understanding these issues is crucial to the approach the system needs to take to break the logjam.

Economics of the Logjam

The essential repetitiveness of the discussion of the information logjam reveals two very important concepts:

- The information that needs to flow in the system should come primarily from the medical knowledge base and the patient record.
- All of the system's stakeholders—providers, educators and students, researchers, consumers, planners and policy makers, and third-party payers—need essentially the same information, but in different forms and at different times and places.

This means that it is possible for information to be collected or created only once and then communicated to meet multiple needs.

In the present system, the burden of trying to achieve adequate information flow for case management, educational reform, research, cost control, and systemwide planning and management is too expensive to even contemplate. If information could be collected or created only once and then shared, however, the economics would shift dramatically in favor of "information liberation."

Systemwide Coordination

While any element or group of elements in the health care system can make the commitment to change, breaking the logjam will require the coordinated action of all elements of the system. That is why an infrastructure that provides a framework for systemwide decision making, planning, and implementation is so essential. For instance, the medical schools cannot remedy their own information logjam without the full cooperation of at least those responsible on a systemwide basis for maintenance of the medical knowledge base, the design of the patient record, and the dissemination network.

It must be kept in mind that lack of information flow is more than just an issue of cost or access; it also stems from an institutionalized mind-set toward preserving the status quo. This attitude is just as important a problem to "solve" as the technological and logistical ones. While information flow alone cannot solve the problems of health care, neither can its problems be solved until the information logjam is broken.

Chapter Six

Information-Liberated Health Care

The health care system is information rich. It has hundreds of millions of patient records, thousands of different textbooks, hundreds of different periodicals, and several on-line information services ranging from hot lines to MEDLINE. Health-related trade publications and articles in magazines and newspapers are ubiquitous. Yet we have seen that too much of the information is of little practical use, relative to its potential, for a wide variety of reasons. Though the system is information rich, it is not information liberated.

In an information-liberated system, information of all kinds would be available to those stakeholders who want or need it, and all parts of the system would create and communicate information freely and appropriately. Let's look at the contrast between the negative scenarios of previous chapters and the positive scenarios of a reformed information system.

Information Liberation
and the Clinical Environment

In an information-liberated system, physicians would have much greater control over their practices and the care they give their patients. They would no longer be victimized by an onerous clerical burden imposed by a bizarre system of third-party billing requirements or frustrated because patient or research information was not at hand.

Case and Practice Management

A unified billing system would be in place, thus greatly simplifying practice management and reducing practice costs. The previous prohibitively time-consuming task of monitoring preventive care would become routine. A very different kind of patient record—something like a spreadsheet—would give physicians the capability to assess at any time the status of any or all patients with respect to such routine matters as preventive care, tests pending, follow-up needed, education planned, or visits not scheduled.

Because all aspects of the patient's complete, high-quality health record, even for care received at other institutions, would be available, repetitive testing and history taking would be unnecessary. Information in the record could be easily analyzed to assist the physician in a variety of useful ways, both individually and collectively. Consultations with distant colleagues and patients would be so easy and beneficial that they would become routine.

A much greater degree of ongoing communication and interaction with patients would take place routinely. Physicians would be able to monitor patients under active treatment more thoroughly. They would be able not only to issue reminders to patients, or clients, for routine screening and preventive care such as vaccinations but also to follow up on those reminders to ensure that the work was done and that the results were communicated appropriately.

Patient education is a key element of sound practice management that would be a big beneficiary of improved information flow. Providers would have the tools and procedures to routinely teach healthy patients about wellness, assist sick patients to play an appropriate role in decision making, and prepare patients and their families for posttreatment self-care.

Inpatient Management

The voluminous inpatient record in its new, multidimensional spreadsheet form would work much harder for caregivers than it does today. Their decision making would be enhanced by their ability to analyze the patient record easily and quickly, and in multiple dimensions, such as over time or across departments. Caregivers would also be able to obtain guidance by analyzing on the spot multiple records of similar cases at the same institution. Individualized care plans and critical pathways developed by nurses would become the norm.

Today it is a tedious task to bring ever-changing information about institutional guidelines and costs to bear on a particular case. But this information could easily be integrated with the patient record as needed, for the further guidance of physician decision making. Moreover, if medical knowledge were liberated, the relevant knowledge, standards, and guidelines could be compared directly and routinely to information in the patient record, thus making the record even more useful.

Medical Knowledge

In the information-liberated system, physicians would no longer have to wonder whether the information they had just read or could recall was really the most definitive. They would have at their fingertips current information about problems they would be likely to encounter in their practices. New information would already be integrated with old information, and both would include not only new medical findings but public health and environmental or industrial factors that might affect their decision making.

Under information liberation, physicians' most valued attribute would no longer be the fund of stored knowledge—their memory—that they must of necessity rely on today. Instead, it would be their ability to bring information resources to bear effectively on specific patient problems.

Physicians would no longer have to wonder just how research findings applied to a particular problem. They would be able to obtain immediate expert assistance with the problem in the office, hospital, or classroom. The assistance could range from information and guidance to standards and advice. Overtech would effectively be prevented, and malpractice claims would be settled by professional arbitration rather than in the courtroom.

Just how far might information liberation be able to take

the clinical environment? Presently, depending on the speciality, a physician might classify a presenting patient into, say, one of one hundred different disease categories with which he or she is familiar. As disease processes became better understood and medical knowledge became more organized and analyzed through information liberation, the number of disease categories and subcategories would be constantly increasing, with fewer and fewer people per category. Eventually, it would almost be possible to have a customized diagnosis for each presenting problem. The next step would be to have customized therapies for each patient as well.

Information Liberation and Medical Education

With the liberation of information, the medical education system would offer instruction aimed directly at creating the kinds of health professionals needed. Information liberation would help to define those needs, and it would help to meet those needs.

Defining the Needs

If information were liberated throughout the health care system, educational planners and policy makers would have access to statistics that would reflect the needs of the population for professionals who would deliver health care. They would also have access to the medical knowledge base, including timely research findings. These planners and policy makers would therefore be able to determine what kinds of graduates would be needed and what kind of educational experiences the students would need in preparation.

Meeting the Needs

If medical knowledge were readily and reliably available in a useful form, the skills physicians would need to practice successfully would be different. The character of medical education would change as well.

Medical students would no longer need to devote so much of their time to memorization; medical education would focus more and more on preparing physicians for careers that heavily involve the skills of information acquisition, use, and management; clinical research; lifelong learning; and decision making. Physicians, themselves liberated from the tyranny of the knowledge base they have had to master, would be able to give their primary attention to their patients' real needs.

The clinical years of medical school, internship, and residency would be very different as clinical medicine became more scholarly. Patients at institutions with residency training programs would no longer have reason to fear the ministrations of residents. Rather than learning by apprenticeship and trial and error, students would learn the bulk of their medical decision-making skills by using training aids, such as simulated patient encounters, based on integrated medical knowledge and information from existing patient records. Because this kind of learning could take place anywhere, students would be able to experience a much wider range of practice environments during their clinical years.

Information Liberation and Research

The process, priorities, and settings of research would change or expand into new arenas with information liberation.

The process of research itself would be greatly enriched in several ways. The patient record would no longer be a barren resource because the high-quality information already collected for that record would become widely available and widely used. Much costly human research could be avoided by first using patient record information and then using simulation techniques to conduct specific research suggested by findings in patient records. Researchers would have much greater access to refined indexes, abstracts, and full texts of publications. As more and more research became systemwide, researchers would be able to collaborate and communicate much more often and freely about research in progress and even about pre-research ideas.

Systemwide research priorities could be set according to systemwide need because communication and information flow would allow those needs to be accurately determined. Research in health care today is overwhelmingly disease based, but other approaches and philosophies would be possible in the future. For instance, health care policy makers and stakeholders might decide to give priority to research that would help use existing medical knowledge rather than create new knowledge. Similarly, priority might be given to developing a better patient record or to public health and wellness research. Costly

117

duplication and unpromising avenues of research would be more easily predicted and avoided.

In addition, if information were liberated, many aspects of research would become routine clinical activities. First, the patient record would be used routinely as a source of research information in either the practice or institution where it is collected and for interinstitutional research. Meticulous attention to high-quality collection and recording of information at all times would be the norm. Second, caregivers and managers would have the skills to research their own records routinely, to answer practice- or institution-specific research questions. Third, the routine use of research findings from many sources would be an essential element of clinical care and practice management, and reliance on memory would fall into disfavor as a sound way to do business.

Finally, if the health care system were to become more cohesive through a bond of information flow and more were known about it as a system, it would not be necessary to "experiment" with the system, thereby avoiding great expense and the risk of disrupting the orderly process of patient care. For example, instead of conducting a statewide or regional experiment to evaluate a new mode of service delivery or a new payment mechanism, researchers could assess the consequences of the new mode or mechanism by carrying out the experiment in a simulated system.

Information Liberation and Consumers

The big winners in an information-liberated health care system would be consumers. They would no longer be expected to take responsibility for their own health in a vacuum of ignorance about health and disease, using only the largely unhelpful and confusing information and mis-information available today. Necessary information re-sources and tools would be available to consumers, and the skills and motivation to use them for personal health management would be part of the standard school cur-riculum.

Consumers would have access to the same medical knowledge base that would be used by the medical com-munity, including information about specific symptoms, diseases, treatments, drug therapies, and outcomes. Moreover, the information would be available in a use-ful and understandable format at convenient times and places.

Consumers would also have ready access to compre-hensive and authoritative information and communication that would promote wellness. Lifestyle information tailored to individual situations and needs would be as accessible and appropriate as the morning paper; so, too, would be updates on the latest medical and wellness research, pub-lic health advisories, and environmental and industrial alerts. In-depth information about health matters of par-ticular interest would also be routinely presented.

Similarly, background information on caregivers and institutions would be available to consumers. Information about caregivers in their community would include edu-cation, practice type, patient-care philosophy, fee sched-ule, and experience with specific types of problems. In-formation about institutions in the community would include an assessment of quality of care, as well as more factual matters such as special facilities and expertise of its medical staff. Consumers would then be able to select compatible providers who have the expertise and experience the consumers want or need. People with special needs that could not be met within the community would be able to obtain similar information about providers in other areas, such as at major medical centers.

Individual consumers would also be able to monitor and maintain their own health record, including information about personal health status, health-related problems, and medical attention received. The record would also contain individualized information about preventive care scheduling, and it could flag certain events and recommended actions. For instance, blood pressure over time could be routinely compared against a threshold that would trigger a suggestion to visit their primary care provider. Any information in the record could be made available selectively to any provider.

Finally, the very personal decisions about how to die and whether to help one's very sick infant live are currently too often made by caregivers or administrators or third-party payers—strangers all. With information liberation, however, consumers of health care would be able to, and expected to, make their own informed decisions about the beginning and end of life for themselves and their loved ones. Specific information about prognosis and the financial and human costs of each option would be available to them. Consumers could then integrate this information with their own values to make such decisions better than anyone else could.

Information Liberation
and Third-Party Payers

Uniform billing would be universal and paying for health care would be demystified because both relative cost and true cost to treat problems would be known. Opportunities for payers to achieve cost savings could be clearly identified, and communication among all stakeholders would be quick and easy.

Insurers and other payers would no longer have to make arbitrary decisions about paying for care. Provider, patient, and payer would have access to the same information about efficacy, safety, side effects, outcomes, and cost of treatment, the information on which such decisions are based. Guidelines would be universally available and applied, but providers or patients would have recourse to arbitration.

Information Liberation and
the Extra-Clinical Environment

Liberated information flow in the health care system would have implications far beyond the clinical uses of information. The system would no longer need to accept the unrestrained growth of unneeded resources or experience the pain of people's unfulfilled health care needs. What is more, it could take responsibility for acquiring information from outside the system to help it meet its goals. Let's look at some examples.

Regional planning for the appropriate number and kind of health facilities and personnel has been difficult. It requires matching information about current and projected health care resources with demographic information about the region and projections about what the region's health care needs will be in the future. With information liberation and communication, such analyses would be routine. In fact, various models for containing unnecessary growth and providing needed facilities and personnel could be considered and priced by means of simulation techniques; planners would no longer have to experiment on the region itself.

Another example involves environmental and industrial surveillance. All too often the insidious effects of pollution, such as an increased incidence of birth defects or cancer, must reach nearly epidemic proportions before they are noticed. If patient records over a given geographic area could be routinely monitored in the aggregate, even very small trends could be detected and investigated through correlation with environmental and industrial information about possible causes.

A third example of reaching beyond the health care system for information pertains to national health status. If the resources of the health care system were no longer being overwhelmed by the tyranny of more information than it can reasonably process and less medical knowledge than it needs, it would be free to devote its resources more fully to understanding and ensuring the health status of the nation. The health care system would be able to communicate readily with other social systems such as education, welfare, and the judiciary and work cooperatively with them to solve common health-related problems.

These might be problems caused by poor health or health knowledge, such as teen pregnancy and failure to do well in school. Or they might be problems that are causes of poor health, such as poverty and substance abuse. Of special concern is the prospect of newly significant infectious diseases and an increase in the incidence of old ones. With better information, communication, and education, the link between the health care system and the public's health could be and must be restored.

An Infrastructure for Information Liberation

To achieve information liberation, the health care system must have an infrastructure. Therefore, stakeholder elements of the system must make a conscious choice to shift their primary locus of concern from their own particular interests to those of the system as a whole. With such an infrastructure, communication of information from one stakeholder or element of the system to another would be legitimized and facilitated. Information would flow in several directions, as described in the following examples.

Localized Flow

Disparate stakeholders at the local level would share appropriate information in the information-liberated health care system. For instance, patients, doctors, and hospitals would share a single health record; local public health planning groups would correlate environmental and industrial pollution information with variations in types of hospital admissions; patient education would become a reality.

Upward Flow

Regions, states, and diverse national organizations would use upward-flowing information from the local level for planning, research, and policy-making. Although this is currently the practice, it is occurring on a very small scale compared to what would be possible if local information were liberated for use throughout the system. For example, it would become routine for specific information from selected patient records to be collected at the local, caregiver level and channeled upward to be used in the aggregate for a national research project sponsored by a professional society or drug company. Thus the local level would contribute to the refinement of the medical knowledge base. As another example, national-level policy makers would use statistics generated at the local level as the basis for refining the mission of educational programs, and regional-level planners might use other statistics for the allocation of scarce regional resources.

Downward Flow

Information would also flow downward. Extensive information, especially medical knowledge-based information and policy guidelines, would be generated at the national level for distribution and use at the local, caregiver level. For instance, authoritative guidelines for the diagnosis and treatment of specific patient problems would be generated and maintained at the national level and made available to all caregivers who wanted and needed them. Public health advisories and organizational changes at the national level would also be communicated downward. Moreover, research information would be readily available in an easy-to-access format for either researchers, clinicians, or consumers.

Thus a health care system infrastructure would cut across and speak for all stakeholders as they worked toward their common mission. To manage and facilitate the necessary information flow, that infrastructure would need to conceptualize an *information framework* that would explain and control the flow of information. Such a framework would define and set criteria for information creation, communication, and utilization within the system. This kind of framework is essential both for achieving the mission of the system and for setting policy in the system.

The information framework described here is not, of course, a concrete, physical entity; it is a concept and a commitment to a common understanding of the way things ought to work and why. More specifically, it is a set of ideas, motivations, goals, and designs that give guidance as to how information should be created, communicated, and used. From the guidance offered by the framework, the actual implementation of its ideas and designs can be carried out.

Chapter Seven

A New Framework
for Information

The task of this chapter is to describe the key concepts
and guidelines for structuring a health information framework and to suggest the conceptual design features it
should contain. However, any consideration of a paradigm
shift on the scale of an information framework for health
care should first take into account what motivations might
persuade those who could collectively make it happen to
actually get involved.

Motivation to Lead

There are several compelling reasons why health care
professionals might want to pursue the idea of an information framework. In each case, the point is made that
participation of health care stakeholders, and especially
health care professionals, is essential, if the system's problems are to be solved.

Fulfillment of Mission

When the system tries to assure better access and high-
quality health care in the face of intensifying cost contain-

ment pressures, it is between a rock and a hard place. Lacking better information on which to base further cost savings, it is not possible for providers to maintain the same level of service with less revenue. The complexity of the dilemma is not well understood even within the health care system. Most "solutions" to health care problems and most approaches to meeting the system's goals have been and continue to be piecemeal.

Partial solutions must be in congruence with all aspects of the health care system's goals, not contradictory to those goals and to each other. While the objective of each partial solution may be worthy in and of itself, each is flawed and creates dissonance in the system to the extent that the action is contrary to key goals. This is typical of most proposed solutions that have been developed in isolation from the goals of both the total system and other stakeholders. For instance, proposals to improve access or provide for long-term care clearly will cost more money than we can afford; proposals to reform the malpractice system might save money, but they could seriously jeopardize quality of care; proposals to save money by paying providers less will inevitably lead to cuts in service; and proposals that permit protection of profits in one area raise the overall cost of care.

It should be clear that the solutions we need are those that take into account and address all parts of the problem at the same time. But this is not likely when external policy makers do not understand the system very well. Proposals that come from *within* the health care system generally do not take into account the mission of the system either. It is important to note, however, that unless and

127

until an information framework is in place, as well as an infrastructure within which stakeholders can take cooperative action, there will be no sound basis for knowing how to propose and take effective action against the system's problems and fulfill its mission.

Cost Containment

Most people understand how to cut administrative costs, and most providers have done so, to the extent possible, on an institution by institution basis. On a systemwide basis, further administrative savings are possible in areas such as uniform billing, malpractice reform, and profit making. However, achieving these further savings requires cooperative agreement and action by all stakeholders.

The other major area where costs can be cut is in physician decision making, but such cost cutting is already posing a threat to quality of care. It is true that what physicians should or should not do in any given case is not always clear, and unnecessary work is sometimes ordered. Physicians' decisions are not always understood even by physicians, and certainly not by patients, policy makers, and third-party payers. Yet in the absence of better clinical guidance, interference in the physician-patient relationship is often arbitrary. This is not an acceptable solution to rising costs, even in the short term.

It has been postulated that there is plenty of money flowing into the health care system, enough to provide high-quality care to all Americans. If this is true, then cost savings in the current way the system does business must come from the health care as well as the administrative areas. There are two essential approaches to meeting this challenge:

- The system needs to better understand how to keep people healthy and out of the system.
- The system needs to learn more about how to care appropriately for people who have entered the system.

Both of these approaches go to the matter of the costs incurred by physicians' decisions. That is, until we have a lot more information than we do now about how to keep people out of the system and how to define and achieve desirable outcomes when they are in the system, we do not have much of a medical basis for further cost containment. Those approaches that lead to cooperative action and improved information flow must therefore precede achievement of the cost containment that could free up resources for greater access and preserve high-quality care.

Health Policy

Because the health care system lacks an infrastructure empowered to make and implement or enforce health policy and an information framework on which to base policy, the perception is that the system is not in charge of its own future. Enforceable policy decisions tend to come from outside the system—primarily from third-party payers and the U.S. Congress. Unfortunately, these policies have been shown to be too often arbitrary and inappropriate, leading to dissonance within the system. They are based

129

on a poor understanding of how the system should operate and what its goal-directed needs are—information that just isn't available.

Health policy decisions regarding organization, financing, research, education, public health, technology assessment, and clinical guidelines should first draw information from throughout the system because policy decisions in one area would have implications for the others. This surely indicates a need for good information and communication, products of an information framework.

As the health care system continues to grow in complexity, it will become even more difficult for external policy makers to make good decisions about health care. This applies equally to the stakeholders in the system. Physicians, hospitals, third-party payers, and pharmaceutical manufacturers are but a few of the groups that understand from personal experience the threat posed by outside regulation and reform. And as consumers try to pay for more and more well-intentioned legislation, they too will begin to wonder why the health care system does not heal itself.

Information is the key, and systemwide information flow is the tool. With an information framework and an infrastructure, the system would have the capability to decide its own destiny. It could plan for implementation of its own goals in its own way. It could plan for and manage its own research, education, policy-making, standard setting, resource acquisition and allocation, and cost control.

An Information Framework as Change Agent

The process of creating an information framework could in itself be the unifying force that would draw major health care stakeholders into cooperative creation of an infrastructure designed to meet their needs on a continuing basis. Each stakeholder has essential information to contribute, and each needs information and communication from the others; collectively their information would have even greater value. As the system learns more about itself, it can achieve a new maturity.

If and when the concepts of an information framework are actually implemented—the subject of later chapters—all stakeholders should also understand that they own a very valuable resource, valuable not only to themselves and others in health care but also to social scientists, researchers, and scholars in the United States and throughout the world.

Goals of the Information Framework

We have seen that the health care system needs to begin taking responsibility for its own mission and policies and for solving its own multiple and acute problems of maintaining quality and opening up access while containing costs. These needs in fact establish the goals for an information framework.

- The information framework should facilitate the provision of information and communication in support of the health care system's mission.

131

- The framework should support policy formation within the system.
- The framework should integrate information and tools that support appropriate, medically necessary, and cost-effective care.
- The framework should foster the health orientation of the population so that expensive acute care will seldom be necessary.

Guiding Principles of the Information Framework

An information framework is essential for envisioning how information needs and resources in one part of the system relate to information needs and resources in other parts and how they all fit into the context of the system as a whole. Several guiding principles must underlie the conceptual structure of an information framework.

Goal Consistency

Concepts and goals of the information framework need to be entirely consistent with the goals of the system to provide affordable access to high-quality health care for all. A successful health care system cannot be achieved if it tries to use the pervasive and vital information resource to give higher priority to other goals such as profit taking. To the extent that the system has strayed from its goals, it will have to reorient itself.

Information as a Systemwide Resource

While specific information may belong to a patient or a provider or an institution, there must be a commitment at all levels of health care to the principle that health information is an invaluable systemwide resource. Further, it is a resource that must be exploited systemwide if the health care system is to function effectively.

The most important task of the information framework in the long run would be to promote a common understanding of the mission of the health care system and of how the system must work to fulfill that mission (see Chapter Two). In doing so it would support a health system infrastructure within which health policy could be made and implemented. The alternative is a dysfunctional system that cannot sustain itself and must be replaced.

Further, the wealth of information in the patient record must be made available for research and education, and medical knowledge must be made more usable and distributed more widely. No other single act or combination of acts could have the impact that freeing the information from these sources would have.

Stakeholder Commitment

Since stakeholder goals and activities need to be entirely consistent with the goals of the system as a whole, each element of the system must be concerned about what its role should be in, say, helping with the access problem, the cost problem, and the quality problem. Thus the conceptual structure of the information framework must support the stakeholders' goal-directed work.

Open-Ended Scope

While the information framework must first help solve today's health system problems, it must be open-ended in

133

scope and sufficiently robust to anticipate and provide for information and communication for the future as well.

Quality

For health-related information to have value in clinical settings and in research, education, and policy formation, it must be reliable in all respects. Therefore, the information framework must provide for the collection of high-quality information that takes into account the multiple and diverse uses to which it might be put.

Accessibility

The information framework must provide for ethical and appropriate access to diverse health information from multiple sources for all goal-serving activities—for example, regional and state planning.

Privacy and Ownership

The framework must provide adequate safeguards to protect privacy and to acknowledge ownership of information.

Feedback

The framework must be responsive to feedback about the needs and goals of health care stakeholders and others who might be affected by what the system does.

Goal-Driven Objectives of the Information Framework

The general goals and guiding principles of the information framework just outlined, along with our analysis of the nature of the crisis facing health care today and an understanding of the pressures that continue to work on the system, point to two initial objectives: to facilitate the collection of certain essential information and then to channel it to those who most urgently need it. As information utilization becomes more pervasive and sophisticated, the specific objectives of the information framework will evolve as well.

The first objective focuses on developing the key information *resources:*

- The medical knowledge base
- The patient record
- Outcomes research

The second objective focuses on how the framework can facilitate the key functional *uses* of the information resources:

- Presenting the medical knowledge base
- Integrating the knowledge base and the patient record
- Refocusing medical education
- Promoting wellness
- Supporting a health care system infrastructure

Key Information Resources

Each of the three key information resources to be developed has a special role in the information framework.

Reconceptualizing the Medical Knowledge Base. The medical knowledge base is, like the universe, essentially boundless and not completely knowable. However, it has for the most part been created to assist with health care, and much can be done to make it more useful for that purpose.

It is helpful to think of the knowledge base in different ways for different purposes, and this is a good place to start doing so. First, we are talking about a body of knowledge, which is the science and practice of medicine. Its physical form and location are not important as long as they are accessible. In fact the knowledge base, or pieces of it, may reside in several different locations at once, including libraries or even the heads of physicians. Specifically, one may think of the anatomy knowledge base and the cardiology knowledge base, which would contain everything that is known about those subjects. In this chapter, though, we are making general statements that apply to all medical knowledge or to any subset of it.

The primary ingredient of the knowledge base is the decades of research results that are enshrined in millions of journal articles. To be really useful, new research information must be promptly integrated with existing related information. The knowledge base further needs to contain information about the relationships among elements in it and rules for using the information.

Presently, writers of textbooks, guidelines, and review articles published by professional societies attempt to describe relationships and rules. Because this is traditional and because we see no other options, we have been undisturbed by the notion that different physicians in different places operate according to entirely different sets of rules, depending on which sources they use. They may even be using sources not accessible to anyone else, such as their own remembered experiences and beliefs. Thus for any given subset of medicine, there may be dozens or even hundreds of different rule sets. This system of using medical knowledge raises serious questions. Generally speaking, are all the different decisions equally valid? Do they all constitute "quality" medical care? Or are some physicians practicing substandard medicine?

One of the first tasks in creating an information framework is to reconceptualize the medical knowledge base from essentially a repository of miscellaneous information to a dynamic, constantly improving, cohesive resource that is accessible and helpful to all who need it.

Of course, changing the very orientation of the knowledge base would necessitate changes in incentives and habits throughout the system. It would be helpful if more publishers, for instance, were to begin to see themselves as purveyors of useful, goal-oriented information rather than of books and journals divided up according to who wrote them and when. Then new information could be added to the knowledge base in a more helpful way. Concurrently, research priorities and academic rewards would need to be redirected toward filling gaps in the content, relationships, and uses of the knowledge base.

Even researchers find the knowledge base cumbersome to use. It is generally accepted that obtaining background information occupies a major portion of researchers' time; but this would not necessarily be the case if information were integrated as it entered the knowledge base. In fact, removing the drudgery of research would in all likelihood offer a substantial intellectual springboard for all types of health-related research.

A medical knowledge base organized for clinical use would be a great boon for students who now must learn in their clinical years through apprenticeship supplemented by tedious research. Using such a knowledge base instead of traditional research, medical students and residents would have time to make sense of what they were trying to learn as well as to see patients. Later we will see specifically how this would work.

As consumers are increasingly being expected to take responsibility for their own health, a usefully organized medical knowledge base would be a real boon. Informed patients would make the work of provider-patient decision making much easier. Even though the knowledge base is already available to consumers who know how to get at it, making good use of it is daunting to all but the most determined and desperate of knowledge seekers.

Many groups in addition to consumers interface with physicians but do not know what to expect from them. These groups are as diverse as hospitals, officers of the court, and third-party payers. When physicians disagree among themselves on the best course of action in a particular situation, it is very difficult for hospitals or the judicial system to know to what standards physicians can be held in any but the most extreme cases. As for third-party payers, it is often hard to imagine which authoritative sources they refer to when they review applications for insurance coverage or claim forms for payment.

It is clear that a reconceptualized medical knowledge

base holds the key to many essential changes throughout the system in arenas ranging from medical education to consumer participation to policy formation.

Upgrading the Patient Record. The second key resource of the information framework, the patient record, has been the object of derision for decades, but little has changed as a result. The record has become so complex and difficult to use that a major overhaul is in order. Earlier discussions have indicated how the record could better serve the patient if it were redesigned as a sort of spreadsheet where variables could be recorded and analyzed over time. It would also better serve the patient if it covered his or her entire health history cumulatively and could be correlated with nonmedical information relating to the patient.

Information in the patient record has a direct educational potential that has scarcely been tapped. Physicians and students alike may want to know what the course of other hospital patients similar to theirs was or what their institution's experience with a certain therapy has been. They could find the answers to such questions quickly and easily from individual and aggregated patient records that had been designed with these kinds of purposes in mind.

In contrast to its present limited use beyond the current illness, the information in the future record would be an especially powerful and valuable tool when it can be aggregated with records from other institutions. Thus an important role for the framework is to obtain information compatibility among institutions.

Obtaining Outcomes Research Results. The liberation

of aggregated patient information would have the most impact in research, especially outcomes research. In the past decade, an alarming incidence of variation in the frequency of procedures has been found to exist among physicians, among hospitals, and among geographic regions. The frequency with which an inpatient procedure is performed is relatively easy to measure and record, and it is without a doubt an indicator of the amount of variation— that exists but is harder to measure—in virtually all aspects of medical practice. It would seem that either a great deal of overtech exists, or procedures are not being done that should be, or both. In any case, it is highly unlikely that the probable level of variation is characteristic of generally good medical practice.

At the same time, independent reviews of medical records have revealed that a distressingly high number of procedures, especially expensive high-technology procedures such as bypass surgery, were really unnecessary. Such examination has even showed that some procedures had no demonstrable value at all or in fact could do more harm than good.

These troubling findings, with their implications for quality of care and cost of overtech, point directly to the conclusion that physicians simply do not have the information they need to provide the best medical care.

The reasonable approach selected by most concerned groups was to use the medical knowledge base, including that aspect of it known as experience or expert opinion, to develop guidelines that would be made available to all physicians. It soon became clear that agreement could be reached for only the simplest and most obvious of guidelines. As noted before, the studies in the literature were collectively inadequate to contribute a great deal of guidance, especially for newer technologies.

Many technologies whose appropriate use has been called into question have already been used extensively with patients. Therefore patient records obviously contain a wealth of information that could be used to study the outcomes. The patient information already collected might actually be able to provide answers to research questions on outcome. At a minimum, its analysis would be a valuable contribution to the medical knowledge base, and it could also raise important research questions and help establish research priorities. The scale of patient record use for these kinds of purposes today is minuscule in comparison to the task.

Key Functional Uses of Information

We turn now to the five key uses of the health care system's information resources as they relate to the system's mission.

Presenting the Medical Knowledge Base. While the medical knowledge base should be as definitive as possible, different communities within the health care system need to be able to consult it in different ways for different purposes. The current linear and unchanging format is really suitable only for scholars of medicine. Tools and techniques must be developed to present specific and possibly complex concepts and their extensions in an easily understandable manner and in a way that satisfies the need.

141

For instance, individuals should be able to make an inquiry about a disease process or a differential diagnosis or possible therapies and get a complete range of relevant but not extraneous information that is appropriately and differently presented for a clinician, a student, or a patient.

Integrating the Medical Knowledge Base and the Patient Record. The usefulness of the medical knowledge base and the patient record would be enhanced exponentially if the two were integrated within the information framework. New knowledge derived from information in the patient record could go fairly directly into the medical knowledge base, the knowledge base could make contributions to the patient record, and both could work together to enrich medical decision making, research, and education. Some examples follow.

- *From the record to the knowledge base.* Earlier discussions have suggested that patient records should be the primary source of preliminary information for outcomes research. The latest findings in outcomes research in turn need to be integrated directly and quickly into the medical knowledge base as a contribution to clinical guidelines. Although outcomes research is daunting and exhaustive, the system and the nation have a critical need for it. Until better information exists about what outcomes truly are and until that information is generally known and acted upon by the medical community, overtech will continue to run rampant. Routinely analyzing all patient records for outcomes and rapidly integrating and disseminating the results should allow the system to converge on overtech much more quickly than would otherwise be possible.

Although outcomes researchers generally analyze the patient record for specific measures of outcome, there is much more of value in the record. The incidence of drug reactions and complications and novel approaches to clinical problem solving are examples of other kinds of information that could be harvested from aggregated records and incorporated directly into the medical knowledge base.

- *From the knowledge base to the patient record.* Medical knowledge pertinent to a specific medical problem generally has only one route to the patient: through the recollection of the physician. The information framework should find a way to make relevant medical knowledge an actual part of the record for all providers to use. For instance, contraindicated medications and recommended tests should become a part of the record.

- *The partnership of medical knowledge and the patient record.* Information integration reaches its peak when medical knowledge and patient information can be considered at the same time and place for medical decision making. The best use of the medical knowledge base is made when it is used in the context of the patient problem. The information framework would need to make available to the physician both the relevant subset of medical knowledge and the patient record. The caregiver in the office or hospital would be able to consider the patient's problems, turn to the knowledge base for information, guidelines, standards, or advice and then apply that advice directly in the decision-making process.

143

Refocusing Medical Education. Reference has been made to the value of reorienting the medical knowledge base and the patient record as tools for clinical education. The model for learning today is that the student must gather specified information, memorize it, and see patients who may or may not have problems relevant to the information learned. Unfortunately, this approach has real relevance to the way medicine is practiced in that what the practicing physician knows may or may not be relevant to the presenting problems. Further, neither physicians nor students are likely to have time to pursue often unrewarding research on the patient's problem.

With the new tools available to both clinicians and students, students would simultaneously learn to use the tools and to use the tools for learning. Instead of relying almost totally on memorization of information that might help them care for their patients, they would learn the concepts that would help them bring highly relevant and readily available information directly to bear on patient problems. Facilitating the reorientation of medical education to take full advantage of the availability of reoriented and integrated information is a daunting task; still, it must be a major objective of the information framework.

Promoting Wellness. Many experts believe that the key to cost containment in health care is to keep people healthy and out of the system. This laudable goal is very difficult to attain when the system does not give priority to creating and dispensing authoritative information on how to stay healthy. Moreover, the system does not make it easy for consumers to understand the circumstances under which it is or is not necessary to see a physician.

Although a great deal of health information is published for consumers, it is difficult for them to accept and follow advice about lifestyle changes given in newspapers and magazines when their own family doctors do not give them that advice and when the system offers little in the way of consumer education programs until disease is present. Many consumers naturally come to believe that taking more responsibility for their own health must not be all that important. Consumers could be much better partners in maintaining wellness if they were better informed. Thus one of the tasks of the information framework would be to meet consumer needs for health education and information.

Supporting a System Infrastructure. Perhaps the most critical objective of the information framework is to help create and support the health care system infrastructure within which the goals of the system and of the framework can be met. The framework would bring together the information and the disciplines needed for an understanding of the health care system and how it operates. Here are some examples of the kinds of information the system infrastructure would need and how it would use that information.

A subset of the medical knowledge base would be the repository of system knowledge, such as its goals, history, sociology, the kinds of professionals it has, what its various facilities are, how it works, and what the interrelationships are. These types of information serve as parameters for understanding the system.

Other information vital to the functioning of the infrastructure would be medical and nonmedical variable information from several sources. Examples include information that has been derived from patient records, such as patient demographics, bed occupancy rates, and costs; summary information, such as incidence of diseases; and external information from statistical data bases on regional demographics or industrial accidents. All these kinds of information are needed for planning.

Because health care policy is only relevant in the context of the society it serves, another important source of information is feedback from society as a whole and from other social systems besides health care about their expectations concerning the health care system.

Conceptual Elements of the Information Framework

The health care information framework we have been discussing presents a unified way of looking at the greatly expanded role that information should play in the health care system and how that role could be achieved; it is the concept level at which commitment to ideas occurs prior to implementation. The framework concepts, which are based on the information *resources and needs* of the health care system, define how information should be generated, collected, treated, moved, and used throughout the system. Once these concepts are spelled out and generally accepted, they can then form the basis for information liberation.

The discussion in this section and the next focuses on defining the following conceptual elements of the information framework and the relationships between them:

146

- Information suppliers
- Information users
- Aggregation
- Brokering
- Communication

Let's look at each of these more closely.

Information Suppliers

When the objectives of the framework were first discussed, it was already clear that the information framework would have a role both in obtaining and in using information. That is, the information framework would first need to identify sources of information, facilitate the collection of high-quality information, and then make it available. Those who provide information are called *suppliers*. These could be providers or other groups from within the health care system, or they could be outside suppliers of nonmedical information. For instance, hospitals could supply information from patient records or about their own operations; medical libraries and publishers could supply medical knowledge; the National Center for Health Statistics would be an outside supplier, as would the U.S. Census Bureau if it supplied demographic information. Even individuals could supply information about their own health to the network.

Information Users

The information framework would also have to ensure that those who need information can get it appropriately at the time and place where it is needed. Those who need information are called *users.* The information could be used for research, education, consultation, public health, or policy-making. The specific users might be doctors, nurses, hospitals, clinics, researchers, consumers, libraries, medical schools, government agencies, or Congress.

Aggregation

Interposed between the information suppliers and users is the function of aggregation, an important design component that would make original information more responsive to user needs and requests. When information leaves its source, several things may need to happen before the information can be used by others. Identifiers may need to be removed, or they may need to be added. The information may need to be abstracted, summarized, or reformatted for specific new uses. If a record is to be combined with others from a different source, it may need to be translated into another coding system, subjected to statistical analysis, combined with reference material, or put into tables. These are all examples of aggregating functions that would make information useful to a wider group than just its originators; any one or several processes such as these could happen to any set of information.

Brokering

The brokering function is also interposed between information suppliers and users. Before information can be given to users it must pass through a conceptual filter of appropriateness. This does not mean that there is a single clearinghouse or just one set of rules; rather, it means that although information flows freely, there are safeguards.

The design element of information brokering includes the ethical guidelines, rules, and contracts that protect the privacy and ownership of information and specify how and why the information may be used, under what circumstances, by whom, and at what cost. That is, brokering defines the nature of control over information. Some guidelines, rules, and contracts are obvious and apply throughout the system. An example might be protection of patient identity or a court ruling on who owns certain types of information. However, most of the rules and contracts would probably evolve over time as the need for them becomes clear in specific situations.

Communication

Communication is, of course, a key design element because without it there is no way for information to get from supplier to users. Several means of communication would be needed for the acquisition and dissemination of health care system information, including electronic communication via computer, but the precise form is not relevant to discussions of the framework concept. What is important is that an appropriate means of communication be available in each situation.

The Conceptual Health Information Framework

Figure 7.1 shows a conceptual representation of the health information framework as a network consisting of the five

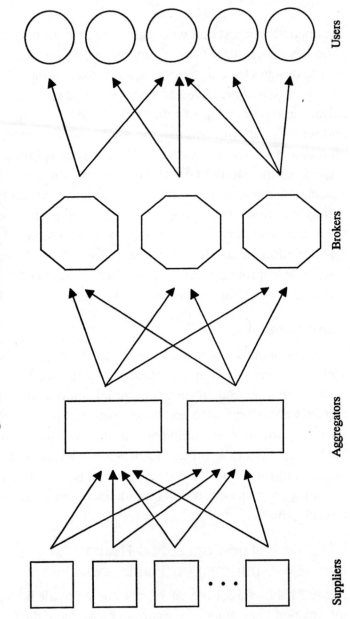

Figure 7.1. Health Information Framework.

Users

Brokers

Aggregators

Suppliers

design elements just identified. Up front, fueling the network, are the suppliers of health information. At the end of the network are the users receiving needed information. Aggregators and brokers are in between, and all are connected by communication links.

It is important to remember that, in this conceptual representation, these design elements may not necessarily be physically distinct entities. For instance, a supplier of information may serve as an aggregator or a broker of information for itself and/or other suppliers. In the simplest example of this, the supplier would send aggregated and brokered information directly to the user.

In the next section we explore the conceptual design elements of the information framework further by applying them to the framework's goal-driven objectives identified earlier in this chapter. It is important to note in each case how well the design elements encompass the three key information resources and their functional uses. To that end, it is useful to think of combinations of these elements as *information flow building blocks* for the information framework; the framework allows us to answer the following questions about the information content of each building block:

Where does it come from?	(Suppliers)
Where does it go?	(Users)
Under what circumstances?	(Aggregation and brokering)
How does it flow?	(Communication)

Design Elements Applied
to Framework Objectives

The initial objectives of the information framework are to develop specific key information resources and to facilitate their use in meeting specific critical information needs in the health care system.

The Medical Knowledge Base

The knowledge base is a valuable information resource that illustrates the applicability of the information framework's conceptual elements. The knowledge base is first a *user* of information from many sources, such as research studies and patient records. Its primary function, however, is that of a *supplier* to those who wish to use the knowledge. It is *aggregated* extensively as new information is evaluated, integrated, and formatted before use. The knowledge base is *brokered* in that in many cases its use is governed by contracts specifying fees that must be paid. Finally, *communication* is an implicit aspect of the knowledge base because information must flow to and from it in some manner.

The Patient Record

In the context of the information framework, the patient record is primarily a *supplier* of information. It could be a *user* of information from other records on the same patient if there were *communication* among records. Because of the scope of the patient record, the information certainly would need to be *aggregated* in some manner, such as by abstraction and summarization. The strict rules governing the ways in which patient records could be accessed and used by others constitute the *brokering* function. Again, *communication* is essential if the record is to have any value beyond its original purpose.

It is worth noting that the patient record is being considered here only in the context of the information framework *for the health care system.* Individual institutions could—and should—define their own information framework, with the patient record at its core.

Outcomes Research

The primary role of outcomes research is fulfilled when it is *supplied* through the medical knowledge base to caregivers in the form of guidance. Outcomes research is also a *user* of information from the patient record and analyses of other records or research studies. The findings of outcomes research are usually public information but are brokered by professional standards for good research. They could be *aggregated* as they are evaluated and integrated with other information in the medical knowledge base. *Communication* is again implicit in disseminating the findings.

Presenting the Knowledge Base

Presenting the knowledge base is first and foremost a task of *aggregation,* as medical knowledge is abstracted, summarized, integrated, and formatted in different ways, according to the needs of various *users.* Appropriate *communication* is also very important.

153

Integrating the Knowledge Base and the Patient Record

Those who want to perform the task of integrating the knowledge base and the patient record would be big *users* of two of health care system's three key information resources. The information they would need from the knowledge base would have been extensively *aggregated*—analyzed, extracted, integrated, and updated. *Brokering* would occur when the users considered professional constraints on comparing the knowledge base directly with information in patient records.

Refocusing Medical Education

Faculty and students would be extensive *users* of *aggregated* information, especially medical knowledge. *Brokering* would consist primarily of the professional considerations that would govern the use of the information in the learning process. In the future, students would be able to use patient records as a tool for learning much more extensively than is possible now, so brokering—ethical, professional, and other guidelines—would be especially important in governing that use. Educational institutions would also *supply* information about the educational process and outcomes back to the health care system.

Promoting Wellness

In meeting consumer needs for health-related education and information, the framework ensures a *supply* of appropriate information from the knowledge base, information especially *aggregated* for the consumer *user. Brokering* would occur at least in contracts setting fees and other conditions for use. Easy and appropriate *communication* is a must if consumer needs for truly useful information are to be met.

Supporting an Infrastructure

In its role as primary policy maker for health care, the health care system infrastructure would be a major *user* of information from throughout the system. As such, *communication* to gather information would be especially important. It would also be important in the dissemination of policy throughout the system and to external systems and subsystems concerned with health policy.

Hypothetical Examples of Information Flow

Thus far the complexity of information flow in health care has been reduced to a framework that is a network of information flow building blocks containing five simple design elements. Let's now consider two information flow scenarios that involve both the design principles of the information framework and the information building blocks. The first example deals with hospital patient records, and the second deals with specialized medical knowledge.

Maxwell Corporation

Maxwell Corporation is a large self-insured corporation that is reviewing regional hospitals' performance on specific quality of care measures the company feels are important indicators. It also wants a database of certain detailed patient information for use with its outcome modeling computer programs. Maxwell engages the Dysart Group, an information service contractor, specifying exactly what information it wants and in what form. Maxwell already has an agreement with regional hospitals specifying that they will provide this information in exchange for payment of the cost of doing so and for consideration by Maxwell as a potential provider to Maxwell's employees. The hospitals have further stipulated that no grouping of fewer than five patients or three doctors per category will be used. The hospitals have done this to further protect the privacy of their patients and staff.

The hospitals remove patient identifiers from their records, add hospital identifiers, and send the information of interest from the required patient subsets to Dysart. Dysart summarizes and analyzes the information and combines all hospitals' information into reports that permit comparison of the hospitals on the parameters specified by Maxwell. It also abstracts and reformats the raw patient information into a database that Maxwell can use to create models of the financial consequences of possible provider-selection decisions. By agreement, the database will self-destruct in sixty days—the amount of time Maxwell believes its decision will take.

In this example the hospitals are suppliers of information from the patient record, and Maxwell Corporation is a user that requires more than one type of information. The hospitals perform some of the aggregating functions, such as adding and/or removing identifiers and extracting only some information from the record instead of sending the entire record to Dysart. Dysart performs extensive aggregating functions, including summarizing, analyzing, abstracting, and reformatting information.

Several instances of brokering occur. Patient and physician privacy are protected not only by removing identifiers but also by not allowing reporting where fewer than five patients or three doctors would be grouped. Contracts between Maxwell and the hospitals and between Maxwell and Dysart stipulate exactly what is to be done, when, by whom, and at what cost. Note that there is no person or agency that can be identified as the "broker"; rather, there is a brokering function, a function that occurs at many points of interface between different elements of the network as appropriate.

The initial information is communicated from the hospitals to Dysart electronically (a computer-to-computer link). Dysart hand delivers its analysis, along with the database on computer disk, and makes an oral presentation to Maxwell, the user.

American Specialists Association

The American Specialists Association owns an extensive library of highly specialized information that members may use free of charge. A physician member in another state calls to request specific information that she needs very quickly. The information involves research and analysis that are beyond the scope of library personnel. On behalf of the physician, the association engages the Library Search Service (LSS), a group of skilled medical library researchers, to fulfill the member's request. The LSS prepares an analysis and supporting portfolio within twenty-four hours, gives the physician an analysis over the telephone or by fax, and sends the portfolio by overnight mail.

The association is the supplier, and the physician is the user. The LSS functions as the aggregator and provides abstracted, summarized, and analyzed information, as well as original articles and reports to back up its analysis.

Once again the brokering function is diffuse but clear. A contract exists between the association and the physician member by virtue of the membership agreement. A contract exists between the association and the LSS as well. There is an unspoken agreement that the association guarantees the quality of the LSS's work by virtue of the association's professional stature.

Communication is accomplished in various appropriate ways. The LSS obtains the research information it needs by using a combination of electronic indexes and abstracts, along with manual searching. It communicates the desired information to the ultimate physician-user first by telephone and then by mail.

Framework Concept Summary

The foregoing examples give some indication of the diverse ways in which users, suppliers, and the aggregating and brokering elements might work together to achieve a goal. A key element has been the many modes of communication used. In both scenarios, some information is transmitted electronically. Other information is conveyed orally (by phone or in person), by fax, or by hand in different forms such as on paper or computer disk.

The point here is that the framework concepts are independent of the mode of communication and, indeed, of the nature of the user, the supplier, the aggregator, and the broker as well. All these elements exist, individually and collectively, for every information transaction.

It is important to keep in mind that the information framework doesn't *do* anything; instead, it is a collection of ideas and guiding principles that must be implemented to achieve the information flow the health care system must have. If the system can implement the ideas in the framework in such a way as to achieve economies of scale, then it can afford to take appropriate—rather than arbitrary—approaches to cost containment, access, and quality of care.

The Role of the Infrastructure

With respect to the information framework, the infrastructure would need to put in place the policies and procedures for achieving information-related objectives concerning content, communication, integration, and implementation.

Information content includes the medical knowledge base, the patient record, and other internal and external information, such as billing, administrative, and demographic information. Only a strong infrastructure can bring about the commitment of all stakeholders to reformulate and maintain the knowledge base and make high-quality patient and other information available.

The responsibility for providing a means of acquisition and dissemination of information must go hand and hand with the task of creation and organization of information.

While accessibility is an objective of the information framework, only a health care infrastructure can make it happen, through the cooperative agreement of all stakeholders who have information to share.

In addition to accessibility of formal information, the communication of informal ideas and information is also important. This form of information flow can be as simple as a telephone call or a face-to-face conversation at a conference. However, because more sophisticated forms of informal communication such as teleconferencing and electronic mail must be available too, an effective infrastructure is needed to facilitate the framework goal of communication as well.

The same system infrastructure must integrate all aspects of the information framework with each other and into the infrastructures of all stakeholders as well. Since a fully achieved information framework has much greater potential than that of the sum of its subordinate functions, full economic, access, and quality benefits can only be attained if no stakeholder continues to operate in isolation. Moreover, the infrastructure has a responsibility for communication and information exchange with elements outside the system that impact health and the use of the health care system. Examples include public health initiatives, national planning such as disaster response that involves health care, and programs that have a health component, such as those that deal with the homeless, drug use, crime, and teen-age dropouts.

Information technology must of necessity play a major role in the implementation of the proposed information framework. The approach taken in this book—to justify the need for information flow first—deliberately puts the computer in the role of assistant to the system's information framework rather than in the role of driver of the framework. The capabilities of information technology—its capacity, its speed, and its ability to mimic the human intellect—go far beyond the mere transmission of information. But if we are waiting for these capabilities to manifest themselves on behalf of health care, we are waiting in vain. They cannot serve the health of Americans unless and until the infrastructure of the health care system leads the way.

Chapter Eight

Harnessing the Power of Information Technology

Thus far we have examined the health care system's desperate need for information liberation, the effects of the existing information logjam, and the value of a carefully conceived information framework within which information liberation could be achieved. However, the scope, complexity, and inefficiency of health care as it is practiced today make it virtually impossible to liberate information successfully within the context of the present system. Thus two dramatic paradigm shifts are essential. First, because the crises in health care are systemwide, only systemwide solutions and commitments can really be effective. A health care system infrastructure that can lead, coordinate, and facilitate change in a way that is compatible with the goals and sociology of the health care system must be created. Second, the sheer volume and complexity of health care information and its flow demand a systemwide commitment, within the context of a system infrastructure, to the extensive, coordinated, and integrated use of information technology.

This chapter explains how information technology has transformed other industries and argues for the appropriateness of information technology as a solution for the health care system as well. It also shows the impact of information technology as a whole on health care and introduces issues related to reliance on the technology.

Lessons from Industry

Information technology is a modern tool for the modern information society. It is no accident that this technology has become highly usable just at the time when the complexities of our society and the scope of its challenges require it. Sheer economic necessity has driven the extensive use of information technology in business and government. The magnitude of their information requirements alone has provided a powerful motivation to introduce the technology.

In the past forty to fifty years many industries have faced information management crises and successfully used information technology to resolve them. Let's look at a few that have solved problems analogous to many of those now facing the health care system.

In the 1950s airlines were faced with larger and faster planes that outstripped their ability to match passenger lists with seat inventory and a host of other information-related problems. American Airlines solved the problem with its computer-based reservations system, which led to its attaining the largest market share of terminal-connected travel agents.

The banking industry faced unmanageable growth in check writing and other banking services, and the attendant escalation of processing and labor costs. With the help of information technology, the Bank of America was the first to use electronic funds transfer to reduce the transit time during which its funds were not available for use, and it sponsored the development of magnetic ink character reading for sorting checks. For many years it led the world in banking automation.

In 1962 American Hospital Supply used information technology to link hospitals directly to its ordering system, establishing itself as the dominant vendor in the industry.

These are just a few of the stories that can be found the absorbing book *Waves of Change: Business Evolution Through Information Technology* (McKenney, 1994), the focus of which is how key visionary and talented managers made it all happen. It was critical to these industries that they develop the ability to process and transport vast quantities of needed information over long distances cheaply, quickly, and reliably. Thus information technology was instrumental—even essential—in revitalizing the industries.

As important as these activities were, by today's standards they were quite limited in scope because their focus was on carrying out already defined activities, simply on a much larger scale. Once the technology was used successfully to mimic existing information-handling processes, visionaries within many industries began to use information strategically, to transform the way they did business. Further, when they were freed from the tyranny of information processing, which had been a formidable drain on resources, they found new ways of interacting with customers and other industries; some even redefined their businesses.

Bank of America went on to use information technology to initiate the massive credit card industry.

The financial industry freed itself from the constraints of time zones when it used information technology to create twenty-four-hour-a-day stock exchanges.

McKenney (1994) points to the dramatic shift in retail business made possible by information technology. The focus moved from budgeting and cost accounting to the more rewarding business of merchandising.

Engineering-based industries, including architecture and aircraft design, were transformed when professionals no longer had to spend a substantial part of their time using slide rules and calculators.

Some industries were fortunate to have been launched in the information age, thus bypassing decades of entrenched policies and procedures that have been rendered obsolete by modern social and technological developments. Two of these are space exploration and the Human Genome Project. Although the possibility of creating these industries had been known, they could not exist as industries without information technology.

What Constitutes Health Care Information Technology?

Computers are used extensively in health care in many exciting ways. Frequently, they are embedded in a piece of equipment or used to control a medical procedure. For example, they are used in equipment that monitors signals from the body, such as heartbeat, respiration rate, and blood pressure, during and after surgery. If any of these signals are outside acceptable limits, an alarm may sound to summon help. Computers also allow physicians to use tomograraphy to peer into the body or guide a cardiac catheter. In addition, computers are a part of many medical laboratory instruments, facilitating highly accurate testing and control.

All these computer applications are involved with creating and using information, but both the creation and the use are immediate, on the human scale. The term *information technology* generally had a much more powerful connotation. It connotes those aspects of computing and communications technology concerned with the creation, storage, manipulation, and flow of information when the intention is the further use of that information; that is, *information technology allows information to have value over time and space*. It includes computer hardware, software, databases—which are files of information—and the means for communication.

Keeping this definition in mind, consider the positive aspects of information technology in health care. Many health care institutional stakeholders have found information technology to be a managerial and cost-controlling boon. Most hospitals have some form of information system in place. Usually, the system is heavily dedicated to financial and managerial needs rather than patient care, but increasingly, the technology is being used as well for communication of patient information while the patient is in the hospital.

The technology has reduced redundant data collection and errors and cut communication delays. It has improved productivity and scheduling. It has improved quality of care through reduction of errors and more efficient information flow. Information technology has facilitated the speed with which research can be conducted and analyzed, and it has had some interesting uses in health-related education. Nevertheless, it is evident that these kinds of uses are not going to move the health care system past its current crises.

To the extent that information technology has had a positive impact on health care, that impact has been where the technology has been used to automate manual procedures, in a manner analogous to its early use by other industries cited at the beginning of the chapter. Further, to the extent that the tools and techniques of the technology are being used in health care, their use is almost exclusively intrainstitutional. One challenge facing health care is to begin transferring these tools and techniques to the system as a whole.

The Economic Power
of Information Technology

Information technology is uniquely suited to the task of reducing the existing scope and complexities of health care information needs to a manageable level. Consider the following characteristics of health care information that make this possible. As we have seen, any given set of information, such as a particular patient record or specific medical knowledge, has many uses throughout the system. For example, a patient record once assembled could be aggregated with other records or other kinds of information and used as a tool for research, education, and planning and as a contributor to the medical knowledge base. Moreover, in most instances, the people and institutions that create or collect information are also the people and institutions that need information. That is, information suppliers are also users. For example, a hospital is a supplier when it furnishes information from the patient record and is a user when it needs information from the knowledge base for its students and the physicians on its staff. Thus we have two fortunate characteristics:

- One information source has multiple uses.
- Suppliers and users are the same people.

So we don't have to treat each information need as a separate, time-consuming, and expensive problem. *The cornerstone of the economic value of the information framework is that a single routine collection of information has a big payoff.* Economies of scale can be achieved with a one-time investment in creating and recording high-quality information and making it available over and over again. Economies of scale can also be achieved when the same mechanisms that deliver information are used to acquire it. It therefore becomes reasonable to think of the information framework as an electronic information network that deals with the drudgery of information liberation, freeing health care professionals to focus sharply on information content and quality.

Sadly, such is not the case today. There are few instances where the use of information technology is being coordinated throughout the system. Having briefly examined the impact of information technology on administrative matters within institutions, let's look now at how modern technology in general and information technology in particular have affected the health care system as a whole.

Technology's Impact on the Health Care System

In a sense, modern technology, especially information technology, is at the root of many of the challenges facing health care today. Were it not for technology, the cottage industry model of forty years ago might still be appropriate. Consider the following examples.

- If the easy availability of high-technology instrumentation such as computed tomography and procedures such as bypass surgery had not occurred, physicians would not have flocked to the specialties in such droves. The array of diagnostic and therapeutic options would be less complex, presenting fewer challenges to physicians' decisions. Clearly, overall health care costs would be lower too.

- Productivity gains in the publishing industry were facilitated by information technology. These in turn have spawned the proliferation of professional books and journals, thus contributing to the information explosion.

- Without information technology, the large databases and the tools for their rapid, complex statistical analysis would not have been available for extensive clinical trials and other large-scale research. The research contributes to the information explosion in health care.

• Without information technology, the extensive outcomes research and meta-analyses being carried out today would be prohibitively difficult. Providers would not be facing the prospect of practicing medicine according to proliferating and doubtless conflicting "guidelines."

• Without information technology, it would not have been possible to administer the Medicare and Medicaid programs because the billing and quality assurance functions could not have been carried out. The cost spiral begun by that legislation would have been delayed.

• Without information technology, the Medicare database could not have been used for the research that has led to prospective payment based on DRGs and to the RBRVS.

• Without information technology to process its claims and compute premiums, the insurance industry could never have transformed itself into the dominant stakeholder it has become.

These examples show how technology—the collective tools, processes, and instrumentation of health care—has been used singularly to advance the science of acute-care medicine through research, development, analysis, and publication. Technology has also been used to extend access to larger and larger groups of people through Medicare.

In some of these cases, however, technology has enabled a different sort of advance: information has been taken from the health care system and used in ways that have caused great dissonance within the system. The DRGs of prospective payment offer one example, and the RBRVS offers another. The beneficiary in each case has not been the system as a whole but selected stakeholders such as payers and their intermediaries.

The collective impact of these kinds of developments has been to shift the focus of health care toward stakeholders' interests and away from the mission and functioning of the larger system. That is, the focus has shifted toward support of specialization, generation of knowledge, and increasingly complex payment algorithms; it has shifted away from the mission of a healthy population that has access to affordable, high-quality health care. As a consequence of existing solely as a collection of stakeholders, the larger system has ceased to evolve. Instead, it has continued to follow the cottage industry model long after this was no longer adequate.

The Health Care System's Dilemma

While the significant developments discussed in the foregoing paragraphs have impacted providers extensively, providers in general were not involved in the decisions leading up to most of these uses of information technology. Now, a window of opportunity exists for the health care system to take control of its own information and use it to develop a more responsive and responsible system. The problems created or exacerbated by the use of information technology can also be ameliorated by information technology—when it is used in a mission-oriented, goal-directed manner.

The impact of technology in general and information technology in particular is indeed powerful, and their use can have both positive and negative consequences. As long as the use of information technology was largely confined to and controlled by individual institutions, its impact was for the most part positive. But integrated use of information across institutions and throughout the health care system acts as a multiplier on impact, as we have seen in the case of the information explosion and in HCFA's use of Medicare data from many institutions to develop DRGs. The key to achieving positive outcomes lies in obtaining the correct locus of control of health information and in the thoughtful provision for use of information technology to maintain that control.

The health care system has no peers when it comes to size and complexity. For size, consider the dimensions of 34 million hospital admissions at over 5,000 institutions occurring each year, along with 1.2 billion office or clinic visits to 500,000 doctors. These visits generate the equivalent of 10 billion pages of medical records per year (Carlone, 1993). In addition, at least that many pages of billing documents must be generated.

The system is highly complex in structure as well, with diverse components ranging from physicians and hospitals to suppliers, payers, researchers, and educators; further, there are few established rules governing roles and relationships. But this diversity pales in complexity when compared to the complexity of the processes of maintaining wellness and delivering care. Considering the size of the health care system, along with its diversity and the complex processes of care, the system almost cannot be understood or described without resorting to the tools of systems theory and, in all likelihood, computer modeling as well.

The health care system has indeed reached the point where its modes of operation border on being no longer adequate to carry out its mission. Its record keeping, managerial capacity, approaches to quality assurance, and mechanisms for planning and policy-making are all straining to keep pace. In fact, the crises in health care are much more far-reaching and complex than those of the industries cited earlier that entered the information age in the 1950s and 1960s. And they will be that much harder to solve. There is no way to turn back the clock to the days of less technology and fewer specialists. The system can only move ahead, adapting to the reality of the times and trying to anticipate future needs. Fortunately, the technology is available to make that possible.

Even within the parameters of current information technology use many gains are possible. A uniform billing system would surely reduce providers' administrative headaches and costs. A computer-based patient record could have an almost immediate impact on health care providers' ability to apply accepted guidelines routinely to patient care. Routine use of patient record information for outcomes research could have a dramatic, relatively immediate impact on overtech.

Even a commitment to these few information technology–based activities would be a significant beginning. But it would be only a beginning. There is still the need for a reconceptualized medical knowledge base, for example, and for all kinds of integrative activities. Nevertheless, the first steps are critical because taking them would mean that the health care system had put in place an infrastructure capable of carrying out systemwide coordination and integration. Once that infrastructure is in place, the door is open for full information liberation.

Health Care System Fears

Another important issue that faces those who would advance the cause of information liberation is the nagging fear of computers that seems to pervade society. This fear goes beyond a generalized fear of technology as something new and different; it goes beyond the fear of being replaced on the job by a computer as well. The greatest fear of health care providers and consumers seems to be a fear of the potential for misuse of health information rather than one of computer-controlled medical tools and techniques.

Consumers have to contend with the social stigma of such health problems as alcoholism, cancer, and mental illness. They also fear the cost implications if it were known that they or a family member might be predisposed to an expensive health problem. They fear that accidental or deliberate disclosure of their family or personal medical history or their current health problems could cost them a promotion or even a job. They could lose or be unable to obtain medical or life insurance. The lives of their family could be disrupted by disclosure of a teen abortion or AIDS. These threats are real in today's health care system, and information technology is perceived as making it easier for information to flow into unfriendly hands.

Providers, too, have seen that the intrusion of information technology makes it easier for others to look over their shoulders. For example, the information that physicians place in the patient record has not changed, but information technology makes it possible for institutions to audit all records, by physician, every day. Physicians are already faced with "economic credentialing" by hospitals. This is the practice whereby "a hospital uses cost/benefit information about a doctor's practice—along with more traditional criteria—in its decision to grant or renew admitting privileges" (Zaldivar, 1993). Economic credentialing could penalize doctors who treat sicker patients, and it could subject physicians to pressure to undertreat in order to save the hospital money.

Physicians are also less than enthusiastic about the proliferation of clinical guidelines. Information technology enables the establishment and dissemination of guidelines, and each institution, plan, and specialty may be expected to develop them. Yet the multiplicity of guidelines is, at least initially, likely to be inadequate and/or conflicting to a troublesome extent. Despite guidelines, physicians still will have good reason to fear more lawsuits and greater loss of autonomy as insurance companies examine every decision physicians make.

At the least, nurses and other health workers may face extensive retraining when information technology is introduced and methods and responsibilities change. Their work can then be more closely monitored and evaluated as well. Worst of all, they fear being replaced by a computer.

Although hospitals make effective use of information technology today, early applications in the 1960s and 1970s saw mostly dismal failures as hospitals tried to implement "total" patient information systems. Still cautious, most hopsitals have ventured only peripherally into patient care systems since then. They also have new reason to be skeptical about the future of automation when it might enable such actions as new kinds of reviews and audits to which they must respond.

Even though these fears and others are justified, this is no reason to reject the technology. On the contrary, such fears add further impetus to the urgent need for the health care system to take control of information technology developments in health care rather than leave them to stakeholders and external policy-making bodies. The sociological consequences of using the technology are just one of the challenges facing designers of the information network.

Chapter Nine

National Health Information System Basics

Now that we have identified the problems, the information framework concepts, and the information technology tools, it is time to begin to formulate an information technology–based solution: the proposed National Health Information System. The NHIS, which would implement the information framework, is presented and discussed only at the conceptual level; the focus is on shaping the health care information framework in a way that would allow it to take best advantage of information technology.

Just as a health care infrastructure must be an integral and integrating part of the health care system, so the information framework should be a part of the health care infrastructure. Further, the NHIS concepts to be described should be considered an integral and integrating part of the information framework (see Figure 9.1), not a separate entity. That is, the NHIS should exist and function solely to serve the goals of the health care system.

It is necessary to develop an understanding of the scope

Figure 9.1. System Relationships.

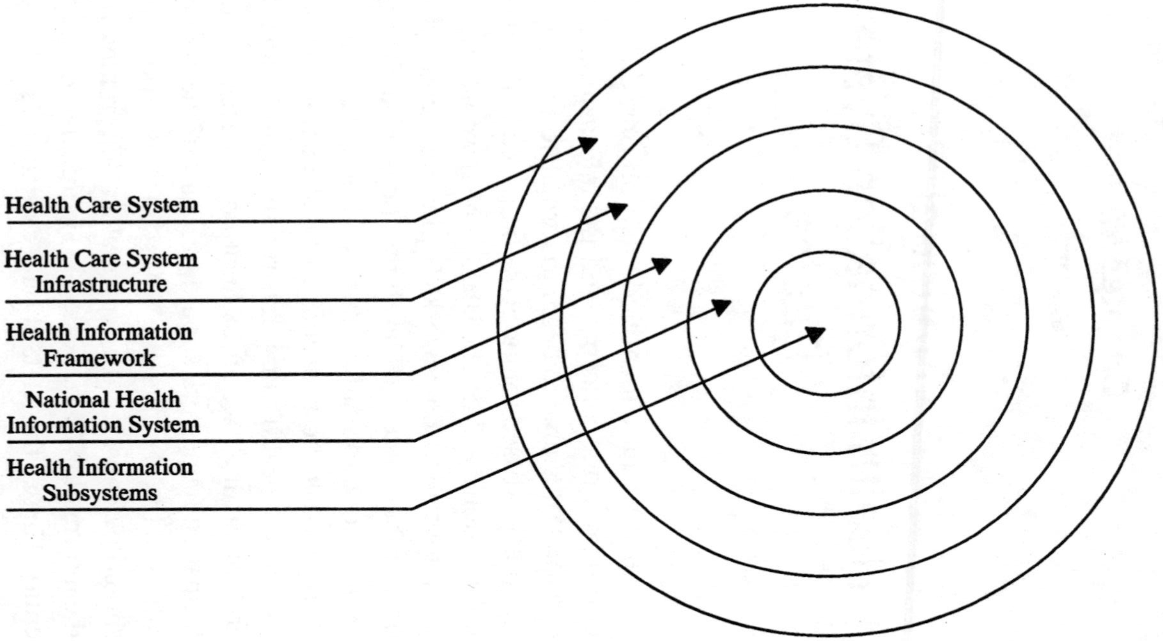

Health Care System

Health Care System
Infrastructure

Health Information
Framework

National Health
Information System

Health Information
Subsystems

of activities that can be supported by the NHIS in order to appreciate fully the benefits of networking and the urgency with which its development must be undertaken. This chapter presents the individual information flow concepts of networking as a prelude to Chapter Ten's discussion of full networks and the issues surrounding their development and use.

Information Flow Building Blocks

Chapter Seven introduced the idea of information flow building blocks, each of which has a specific information purpose and meets a specific information need in the health care system. Each building block has one or more suppliers, one or more users, and aggregation, brokering, and communication functions. The same chapter also suggested that an information framework that would assemble these building blocks into an information flow network could be conceptualized.

This section further describes the universal applicability of information flow building blocks as the basic components of the NHIS. Let's look first at some of the different ways information needs can present themselves. Consider the examples shown in Figure 9.2.

Service Configuration

Figure 9.2 shows the simplest form of transaction, a one-time instance where a supplier gives information to a user. When that supplier's information is well organized and accessible by computer, it is called a *database*. The form in which users receive their subset of the information is called

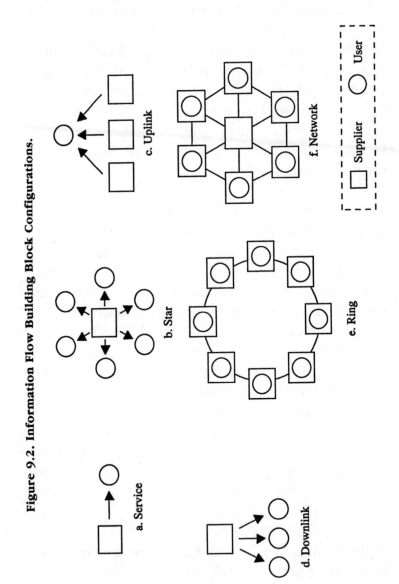

Figure 9.2. Information Flow Building Block Configurations.

the *format*. The supplier is responsible for aggregating, or packaging, the information, and each user is responsible for imposing any brokering standards on the information. An example would be a physician's office sending an order for Xrays to a radiology clinic. In the information sense, the physician is supplying information and the radiology clinic is the user. When the results come back, the roles are reversed. In either case, however, the user functions as broker because it is the user that decides what the need is and whether it has been adequately met.

Star Configuration

In the star configuration, shown in Figure 9.2b, a central source of information directs information to external points. This flow concept might be appropriate when a hospital offers physicians the capability of connecting electronically directly to its medical record database. Thus physicians in their offices or homes could review test results and progress notes in their patients' hospital records. The physicians are the information users, and the hospital is the supplier, aggregator, and broker of information.

The star configuration works as well in reverse: in addition to receiving information from the hospital, physicians could use the same linkage to send information to the hospital to order tests on their patients. In this case, physicians are suppliers, and the hospital is the user, aggregator, and broker. Note that in both cases the hospital is both aggregator and broker. This is because the electronic link would no doubt be defined and established by the hospital and then offered as a service to physicians. The hospital would be responsible for such brokering functions as specifying who could read the information or issue orders and deciding what orders it would accept. It would also be responsible for such aggregating tasks as adding identifiers, verifying user identity, and routing each order to the correct department.

Uplink Configuration

An uplink configuration, shown in Figure 9.2c, is used when a single user needs information from several sources for a specific purpose. Today this configuration is typically used only when required by law or other strong motivating force, such as billing a third-party payer. Voluntary sharing for a common external purpose is currently the exception. Still, this is a common configuration, and it should become even more common.

For example, multi-institutional clinical or health services research projects would use uplinking to collect information from multiple facilities for statistical analysis at a central location. Uplinking would occur when information is collected from multiple providers as part of a regional or national health-planning effort. Information on personnel, facilities, and utilization would be needed to help plan for future funding and distribution of health care–related resources.

Moreover, some instances of updating the medical knowledge base are instances of uplinking. When physicians send information about adverse drug reactions to pharmaceutical companies or notify the Public Health Department about certain cases of communicable disease, they are updating the knowledge base. Currently, new research findings are disseminated directly by agents (publishers) of the suppliers (researchers); however, findings could be aggregated for the knowledge base by means of the uplink configuration.

Since aggregation is a more complex function in the uplink configuration, it may be done by a third party. Companies that receive and process claims for insurance companies are an example. Similarly, the National Library of Medicine acts as aggregator for the medical knowledge base when it acts as a repository for research publications, creates indexes and search strategies, and generally tries to improve user access to research findings.

When the information being supplied involves patients, whether it is billing or clinical, it is typically heavily brokered to ensure its appropriate use. On the other hand, information sent to the knowledge base may not be brokered because it has already been published. As a general rule, when the supplier is required by the user to provide information, more brokering is involved to provide safeguards and to make sure the information is usable. For instance, because billing information is typically required to be supplied in a rigid format, a broad range of formal and informal agreements and professional standards may apply.

Downlink Configuration

The downlink configuration, shown in Figure 9.2d, should enjoy wide application in the future. Virtually all dissemination of information from the medical knowledge base falls in this category. Some examples are public health advisories, patient education programs, and significant new clinical research findings. Eventually, extensive clinical guidance should be available through the use of this configuration.

Because the knowledge base is not a single entity and parts of it may be in entirely different locations, different procedures and rules for access would apply in different situations. Aggregation would be done by suppliers, who would tailor the content and format of the information requested to the specific capabilities and needs of the user. Except for value-added service charges, brokering would not be an issue because health-related information is generally regarded as a public property.

Ring Configuration

The ring configuration, shown in Figure 9.2e, connotes a colleagial relationship in which information is shared by all players. That is, each node on the ring is usually both a user and a supplier, and all the user-suppliers are peers, with little or no hierarchy among them. This configuration concept is very common within institutions where employees have a high need for the same information resources and/or for the same communication routes, such as within companies or hospitals. In hospitals, for instance, virtually all professional and clerical staff members work with and share information in the patient record, and all clinical services need to communicate with ancillary departments such as laboratories. Thus a ring configuration would be appropriate.

However, in keeping with the fragmented and competitive nature of health care today, there is little direct peer sharing of information among institutions or providers other than consultations and referrals. Therefore, the synergy enabled by information sharing among professional peers does not occur. Because this situation should change in the future, the ring configuration will become widely applicable.

The research community offers a good example of the potential for information sharing through a ring configuration. Because researchers have long been accustomed to using computer technology, they have adapted readily to communicating electronically. However, their communication by computer has been largely informal, such as using electronic mail (passing notes) or electronic bulletin boards (announcing conferences or employment opportunities).

Currently, the sociology and politics of health care research do not encourage the sharing of ideas, databases, and findings in advance of publication. An exception is the Human Genome Project, where the scope of the research is too great for any single facility to undertake. Project tools and resources such as databases are spread among many research facilities and accessed by all through the use of information technology. This is in contrast to the multi-institutional research mentioned earlier, where information is collected and delivered through an uplink to a common point for processing and analysis.

Combination Configuration

Many information flow building blocks, representing specific health care information needs, are more complex than the foregoing examples would indicate. For instance, if providers were to begin sharing a common medical record system for everyone in the community, aspects of a ring configuration, where each provider both contributes to and uses information in the record, would come into play. Since the record would in all likelihood be physically housed in a single location, however, the configuration could also be thought of as a star.

Going a step farther, health care providers might decide to use the network for more purposes than sharing the common medical record. The same network mechanisms could facilitate consultation reports, the sharing of educational programs, electronic mail, and electronic bulletin boards. Typically, each user-supplier would offer some special service or function to the others. For instance, one hospital might physically house the common medical record, while another provider might offer educational programs, a third might offer electronic mail and bulletin board services, and a fourth might maintain the physical communication facilities.

Obviously, the arrangements can become quite complex, leading to complex aggregation and brokering functions as well. Since all information does not flow through a common point, each user-supplier could serve as the aggregator as appropriate for the functions and services it provides, according to brokering guidelines agreed upon by all user-suppliers.

Maintaining the medical knowledge base represents another combination configuration. New knowledge may come from researchers' facilities, pharmaceutical companies, providers (from the patient record), or statistical databases (for example, census data). To the extent that professionals voluntarily contribute information to be processed and shared with other professionals, maintaining the medical knowledge base could conceptually be considered a ring configuration. However, because the acquisition of information so dominates the maintenance function, the configuration appears to function as an uplink. In the future, information will flow to the knowledge base as a matter of course, as a by-product of other information-based transactions. Then the focus of maintenance can be shifted to the highly complex but more rewarding functions of analysis and integration of the newly acquired information.

Network Configuration

If extensive employment of information technology is to become at all practical for health care, then several building blocks must be combined effectively and efficiently. That is, the physical computer network must be able to accommodate almost any kind of information need. Figure 9.2f shows a network configuration that accommodates all the other configurations illustrated in Figure 9.2. Close examination should reveal that stars, uplinks, downlinks, and rings are all contained within the single network.

Fortunately for the health care community, information technology is capable of providing all these kinds of linkages simultaneously and in a manner that is undetectable to users and suppliers. Thus health care professionals need give no further consideration to physical linkages. Instead, if these professionals are connected to the NHIS, all these styles of information flow will be available to them. As a result, they will only have to deal with these styles conceptually and only where a particular style is useful to them.

Scope of Information Networking

Information is needed and should be available on many levels. Some information has only institutional or local utility and need not be made available on a wider basis. Other information is best made available and/or used on a regional basis, whereas still other information needs are most effectively met on a national scale.

Because it is important that the NHIS effectively accommodate the scope of all information functions and allocate them properly in the network, health professionals need to consider functional levels in their planning. This section looks at how networks that differ in scope—local, regional, national—are appropriate for different types of functions.

National Level of Information Networking

Americans expect to receive the same high quality of health care wherever they go in the United States. In this era of personal mobility, instant communication, and concern for fairness, there is every reason for health care to be consistently delivered. Further, many essential functions will have to be needlessly duplicated in each region if they are not coordinated nationally.

Even though activities may most effectively be carried out at a national level, this does *not* necessarily mean that they must be carried out by the federal government. In fact, in most cases it would be more appropriate for agents of the health care system to direct these functions. The kinds of functions best served at the national level are as follows:

- Making health care policies that affect all Americans, such as those regarding access, financing, facilities, personnel, and public health
- Coordinating the maintenance and use of the medical knowledge base
- Developing clinical guidelines that apply equally throughout the country
- Standardizing educational programs, including the development and maintenance of computer-based educational programs for health professionals and consumers
- Collecting and maintaining nonclinical health care information for health care research, education, and policy making, including information about the health status of population groups, personnel, facilities, policies, costs, and public health problems that are national in scope such as crime, substance abuse, outbreaks of infectious diseases, and environmental hazards to health
- Coordinating information resources between federal and other national databases (*The Feasibility of Linking*, 1991)
- Keeping medical records for itinerant and other special populations

- Planning and coordinating health services for national and international disasters
- Maintaining a locator service because information resources will be held in diverse locations throughout the country

All these national-level functions would require extensive use of the NHIS. Those that are being carried out at all today are severely hampered by the information logjam. Besides facilitating coordination, one of the most important services the NHIS would offer in carrying out these functions at the national level would be to act as a communications link between regions of the country and between national agencies and organizations.

Regional Level of Information Networking

Many health care activities, and therefore information functions, are regional in scope (Duncan, 1983). An example of a region might be the San Francisco Bay area or the New England states. Here are several examples of regional-level functions in an information liberated health care system:

- Regional planning and policy-making to determine the need for and optimal allocation of health facilities, personnel, and financing in the region
- Conducting multi-institutional research that requires regional information collection and analysis
- Monitoring environmental and other public health hazards and natural disasters wholly within the region
- Maintaining health-related databases on regional

health status, costs, expenditures, personnel, and facilities

- Creating medical and consumer educational programs specific to the region or population
- Paying for health care because, regardless of payer, in the future the region may well be the most reasonable locus for coordinating and managing a payment system
- Assessing quality of care, including evaluating institutions, maintaining quality records, and monitoring prescriptions for improvement

As is the case with functions at the national level, even these rather obvious regional-level functions are not and cannot be carried out effectively without extensive use of information technology. The most significant information function of the regional level may be to act as a value-added conduit between the local and national levels and between the local facilities and other regions. For example, the regional level may facilitate a downlink for clinical guidelines and education materials from the national level to the local level. At the same time, it may facilitate an uplink for medical records at the local level to the medical knowledge base at the national level. Such activities are discussed in further detail later in this chapter.

Local Level of Information Networking

Information issues *within* provider facilities are critically important, but much has been written about those topics, especially about hospital information systems. This discussion focuses on the *interinstitutional* aspects of local networking. The kinds of information functions best served at the local level include the following:

- Maintaining medical records for a population that receives health care at diverse locations, including the workplace and the home
- Offering consumers full access to the medical knowledge base and to educational programs tailored for their needs
- Monitoring hospital admissions for signs of adverse events that might signal the effects of environmental hazards or an increase in the incidence of an infectious disease
- Maintaining local databases on health status, facilities, personnel, costs, and quality of care
- Coordinating scheduling for patients with multiple providers
- Tracking patient compliance with preventive care schedules, wellness and other educational programs, and treatment plans
- Providing informal communication, consultations, and referrals between providers
- Offering clinicians up-to-date information about educational opportunities, new clinical guidelines, and other research findings, public health bulletins, and summary news and statistics about local health care status, practices, and costs
- Making specialized software available to providers, researchers, and other health care personnel, includ-

ing programs for simulation and modeling that incorporate local demographic and health-related information, programs for scheduling and compliance monitoring, a clinical record framework, specialized database search strategies, access to research databases, and statistical analyses

As is the case at the regional and national levels, these local-level functions are scarcely carried out today. In fact, most would be virtually impossible to carry out effectively, if at all, without using a computer network. In addition to these purely local functions, one of the most important tasks at the local level is to supply a conduit between the providers and the regional and national levels. Such a conduit would be an uplink for the medical record and a downlink for access to products of the medical knowledge base.

Information Service Centers

Today, efforts toward increased use of information technology in health care are focused on building up the medical knowledge base ("Improving Health," 1989) and automating the patient record (Dick and Steen, 1991). However, the foregoing examples of functions appropriate at the national, regional, and local levels show that work on the patient record and the medical knowledge base is just a starting point for the NHIS. The examples above reflect a complex array of diverse kinds of information going in every imaginable direction for a wide variety of purposes. The most difficult tasks for the NHIS are not collecting and transmitting information, however; the most difficult tasks from the viewpoint of the network are *those that make the information useful*—the tasks of aggregation and brokering.

For these tasks, and many others that do not seem to be in the province of individual suppliers and users, the concept of *information service centers* is essential. These would be facilities of all kinds that provide networking services that users and suppliers are not willing or able to provide. Before examining how these might work, let's first look more closely at just what constitutes aggregation and brokering, two of the most important functions of a service center, and then at other functions for which a service center would be useful.

Aggregation

In general, aggregation has been defined as the activities and processes that make information useful to the user. These activities, in no particular order, are some that would apply:

Receive	Compare
Identify	Analyze
Verify	Index/abstract
Separate/collate	Summarize
Encode/decode	Combine/merge
Create/update/	Format/reformat
maintain databases	Label

Brokering

Brokering has been defined as the application of rules that govern the flow of information. Brokering particularly ensures that the user's needs are specified and met and that the supplier's constraints and/or caveats about the use of its information are respected. The rules could specify any or all of the following and more:

Content	What should be collected?
Format	In what form?
Place	Where should it go?
Route	How should it go?
Time	On what schedule?
Duration	For how long?
Conditions of use	For what purpose?
Cost, payer, and payee	Who pays how much to whom?
Compliance/evaluation	Was it done correctly?
Purging	Is the information still needed?

Brokering is not an easy concept to implement. Much health care information would be needed for many different external purposes, each requiring different subsets of the information in different forms and going different places on different schedules. For example, information in the medical record would be needed for research, education, planning, and policy-making. Coordinating all these functions efficiently and effectively would be a brokering task as well.

The brokering function could obtain its guidance from one or more sources, such as these:

Laws

Regulations

Contracts

Memoranda of understanding

Requests

Community standards

Common sense

Religious beliefs

Other Network Functions

Several additional vital network services do not fit neatly into the preceding classification schemes; they may contain elements of each plus an element of communication. Here are some types of services, with examples, that an information service center might perform:

- Locate a user, supplier, software program or other information resource. A provider asks for the location of specialists whom he or she can contact over the network for a consultation on an unusual clinical problem.
- Link functions across regions or communities. Several local medical societies join in conducting grand rounds via videoconferencing facilities.

196

- Pass information through for an uplink or a downlink. Medical record summaries or educational material are transmitted.
- Broadcast or selectively disseminate information. Public health notices are broadcast; information about a drug being tested by several local providers is disseminated solely to those providers.
- Notify users, suppliers, aggregators, and brokers of events. A regional conference on health care reform is scheduled, and continuing education credit is available.
- Remind users and suppliers as requested. Suppliers are notified when information is due to be forwarded; users are reminded when it is time for a previously scheduled electronic conference.
- Monitor information content and flow. Medical records are routinely scanned to detect an increased incidence in certain birth defects in selected neighborhoods, evidence of an increased level of ground water pollution by the Chempol Company.
- Bill a customer for information services. The billing and collection of information service fees are bound to be complex.

It seems clear that there must be a way of providing the many services of aggregation, brokering, and other network functions. If suppliers and users were to communicate directly with one another, the network—and users— would be overwhelmed. Information service centers at every level are the answer (Duncan, 1982, 1983).

Service centers would provide the network with a

powerful concentration of skills, knowledge, and technologies that could free suppliers and users from repetitive and/or complex tasks outside the needs of their own businesses. Figures 9.3, 9.4, and 9.5 show typical information service centers at the national, regional, and local levels. Note that in each case they connect all players at their level as appropriate, and they also connect to the other levels. Thus the idea of service centers makes possible all the networking building blocks shown in Figure 9.2 because it enables combined networks (see Figure 9.2f) to function smoothly despite their complexity.

Multiple information service centers would be needed for each local area or region as well as nationally. Each might be specialized by information function, network function, or political boundary, to name just a few. However, such differences would be transparent to both user and supplier because all service centers would be a part of the same network.

We are now ready to consider how these basic networking ideas can be combined in specialized networks and examine the issues surrounding them.

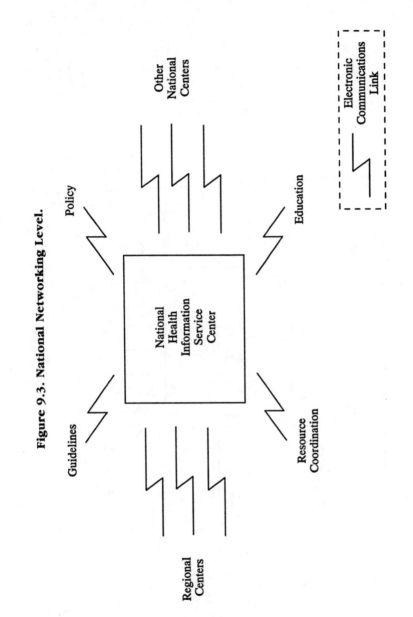

Figure 9.3. National Networking Level.

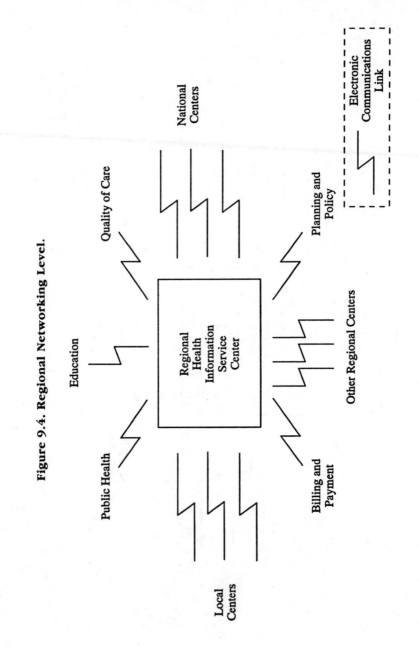

Figure 9.4. Regional Networking Level.

Figure 9.5. Local Networking Level.

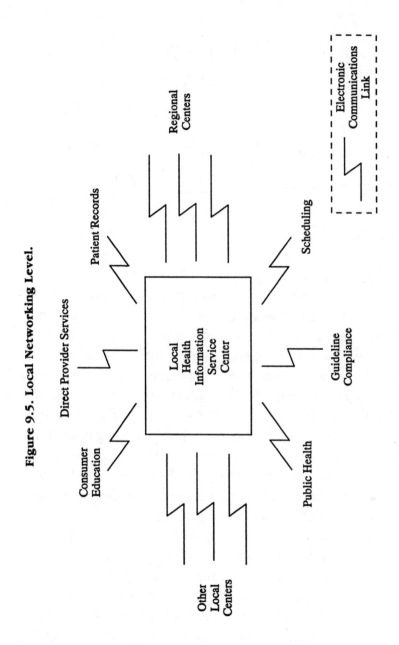

Chapter Ten

Special Purpose Networks for Health Care

Chapter Nine showed how information flow building blocks could exist in several different patterns, depending on their intended function; how different information needs have different geographic scope; and how information service centers could function as a mechanism for carrying out the various tasks of aggregation, brokering, and other network functions. This chapter pulls these various basic ideas together to show how they might work as specialized networks in selected areas of health care to meet important information needs. The hypothetical networks used as examples are national in scope because the information needs are national in scope.

It would be natural in today's health care climate to assume that because some networks are national they must be government networks. But, as noted earlier, that is not the case. Consider such private national organizations as the National Football League, the First National Bank, and American Airlines; clearly, these are not government agencies. As each network in this chapter is considered, readers are asked to imagine that the health care system has already initiated and developed, and now owns/controls, the network and the system it serves.

The notion of specialized networks may suggest that the NHIS is several networks in one, and that would be exactly right conceptually. The information resources and needs of most health care professionals do not encompass the universe of health information but rather a useful subset of it. As we consider the NHIS at increasingly complex levels, it is therefore useful to look at its functions separately, according to such meaningful health care arenas as education, research, and clinical specialty.

Physically, because of the extensive overlap of suppliers' resources and users' needs, a practical and useful NHIS would need to be either a single network or, more likely, a web of interlocking specialized networks. These networks might be specialized according to health care arena, size, geographic scope, or politics. In general, however, the capabilities of communications technology are such that the physical structure of any network would not be a matter for concern in most discussions of health information flow; what is important physically is that health professionals have appropriate and adequate access to that network.

Looking at the NHIS by arena is not an attempt to simplify the complexity of the information flow problem in health care, an all too common exercise. Rather, it is a realistic and practical way to show how the basic elements of an NHIS combine to carry out important health care func-

203

tions. The examples that follow include just enough detail to be illustrative and are not meant to depict *all* the desirable functions in their particular arena. Again, these examples are based on the assumption that the health care infrastructure and information framework are already in place.

National Clinical Guidelines Information System

The National Clinical Guidelines Information System, also referred to as the Guidelines System, is responsible for the development and dissemination of guidelines for clinical practice. It is a hypothetical system developed in response to the overwhelming need of practitioners for help in coping with the quantities of new and often conflicting clinical information. Figure 10.1 shows the Guidelines System network, which will facilitate the system's work. Let's take a closer look at the elements of this system and its network.

National Clinical Guidelines Center

At the heart of the Guidelines System is an information service center, the National Clinical Guidelines Center, informally called the Guidelines Center. There, new information is gathered, analyzed, and integrated with existing information, and the resulting guidelines are disseminated.

For the whole of medicine, millions of guidelines will be needed. The first set of guidelines will be the product of the labor of thousands of physicians and scientists working for several years. The pace of research being what it is today, many guidelines will become outdated almost as

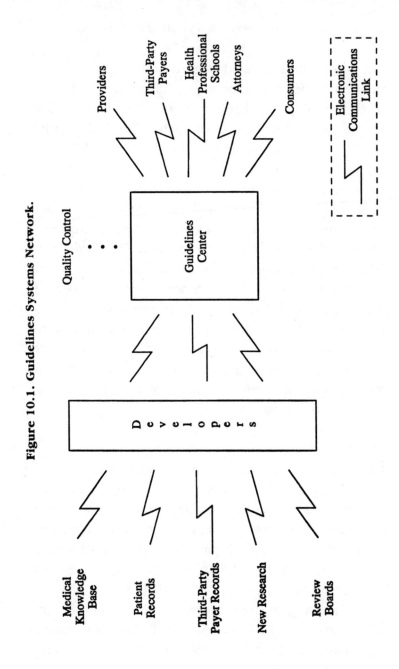

Figure 10.1. Guidelines Systems Network.

fast as they are issued, so hundreds of people will continue to work on keeping the guidelines updated.

Of course, these people will not all be in one place. In fact, every medical center, research facility, and specialty board in the country will have formal responsibility for maintaining guidelines in selected areas. The National Cholesterol Education Program Panel on Detection, Evaluation, and Treatment of High Blood Cholesterol in Adults, which issues recommendations for blood cholesterol management (National Cholesterol Education Program, 1993) offers an example of how specialists and scholars might contribute to the guidelines. Since all the developers of this program are connected to the same high-powered electronic network as the Guidelines Center is, they really cannot tell whether their colleagues are in the next room or the next state. The functions of the Guidelines Center in development are therefore those of coordination, administration, and management.

Suppliers

Guideline developers in each clinical area will use several sources to establish the guidelines initially. As indicated in Figure 10.1, among the most important of these are the existing medical knowledge base, patient records (privacy protected), and third-party payer records, all of which are available through the NHIS. In many cases new outcomes research studies, including clinical trials, will be ordered to supplement existing information. All this information will be analyzed and its essence distilled into guidelines. The Guidelines Center will possess not only the guidelines but also the extensive treatises on which the guidelines in each clinical area are based. These treatises, which can be accessed electronically, are called collectively the Guideline Background Databases. As new research or other information (such as adverse drug reactions) becomes available, it will be verified and integrated with the information already in those databases; then the guidelines themselves will be updated.

Aggregation

Several levels and types of resource aggregation will occur. Before the medical knowledge base ever reaches the Guidelines Center or its satellite developers, those aspects of it that are housed at the National Library of Medicine will already be indexed and abstracted. Individual developers will further aggregate by acquiring and analyzing information from the medical knowledge base and other sources and then forwarding it to the Guidelines Center. The center itself will verify the guidelines it receives from developers and then package them in usable units for dissemination.

Brokering

Most brokering functions—specification of content, format, place, route, time, duration, conditions of use, and cost—will be managed by the Guidelines Center in its role of coordinator of the entire specialty system. Typically, the costs of maintaining the system will be covered by user fees for network and information use. These fees will be collected by the center or its agent.

Users

Individual providers, provider institutions, and other health care stakeholders such as third-party payers, attorneys, health professional schools, and consumers will use the guidelines directly or indirectly.

Other System Functions

The Guidelines Center or its agent, such as the U.S. Postal Service, or the NHIS overall network, will actually disseminate the guidelines, according to the brokering agreements. Here are two scenarios. Institutions or individuals may subscribe to receive an updated customized, computer-readable compact disc every quarter. The disc will contain the latest guidelines in clinical areas the subscriber has specified. Alternatively, guidelines may be maintained in a central database to which subscribers can connect through their own computers. The possibility also exists that extensive additional uses can be made of the end products and by-products of the guidelines work (as the example for medical education illustrates).

Information Framework Criteria for Success

In Chapter Seven, important information framework criteria in the form of guiding principles, goals, and objectives were spelled out. Since the NHIS represents the implementation of the information framework and since the Guidelines System is a subset of the NHIS, the Guidelines System design must—and does indeed—meet these framework criteria for a "good" health information system:

- Clearly defined system elements and functions
- Goal orientation
- Information as a systemwide resource
- Stakeholder commitment
- Open-ended scope
- Quality (verification)
- Accessibility
- Privacy and ownership
- Responsiveness to feedback
- Support of system's mission
- Support of policy formation
- Support of appropriate care
- Use of existing information resources
- Presentation of medical knowledge
- Integration of the medical knowledge base and patient record
- Aid to medical education
- Support of health care infrastructure

National Health Education Information System

Once the medical education establishment has recognized that its graduates spend most of their professional lives behind the information curve, and after it has formulated guideline-oriented curricular changes, it then faces the task of generating, maintaining, and providing access to new teaching materials. Information technology will be essential in implementing any new curriculum, so the hypothetical National Health Education Information System, also known here as the Education System, will be a central player. The Education System network is shown in Figure 10.2. Let's look at the components of the system and its network and see how they function together.

National Health
Educational Development Center

Developing educational materials is a very expensive process. To avoid redundant development and to produce equally skilled graduates throughout the country, the National Health Educational Development Center, or Education Center, is designed to coordinate the development, maintenance, and distribution of educational materials. To minimize costs through sharing, nursing and other health professional education groups will be invited to participate. The medical knowledge that various students should have will be divided up according to clinical area and level (depth) of knowledge needed.

As is the case with the Guidelines Center, development of content and pedagogy will be spread across the country among dozens of academic centers and research groups connected to the Education Center by the Education System network. Much of the work will be done by faculty members, thus meeting the need to reorient faculty at the time development is taking place. The Education Center will assume a larger role than the Guidelines Center in the actual development because a wider range of professional skills is needed for developing educational programs than for creating clinical guidelines. That is, professional educators, cognitive scientists, and computer scientists are also needed to create computer-based multimedia learning materials.

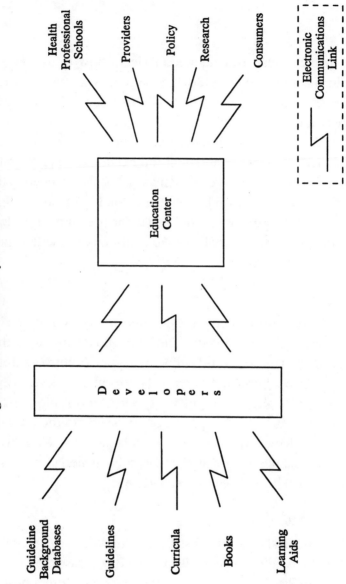

Figure 10.2. Education System Network.

Suppliers

Since medical students need to learn how to use guidelines in practice, the guidelines and delivery mechanisms developed by the Guidelines System will be made directly available to health professional schools. However, students need to know much more about the hows and whys of clinical approaches and decision making than just the final decision, so more basic material is also needed. The most useful tool will be the Guideline Background Databases that describe the rationales for the guidelines. Existing learning materials such as textbooks and videotapes will be used as well.

Aggregation

The Education Center will acquire its needed materials primarily by receiving the guidelines and databases via the Education System's and Guideline System's network linkages. The Education Center will perform extensive analysis, design, and development at its various locations. The materials will then be packaged according to the level of knowledge needed about a particular subject. Whenever the guidelines are updated, the learning materials will also be updated on a realistic schedule.

Brokering

The medical education establishment will obtain permission to use the Guideline Background Databases and share its own development costs and products with other health professional education groups. These are good examples of brokering in advance of forming a network, which can be done if there is an infrastructure in place with the authority and ability to take such actions. The synergy is clear because these actions will allow the guideline developers to recoup some of their development costs as well.

Brokering functions regarding the use of developed programs will be carried out by the Education Center, which will always be eager to find new ways of sharing information and costs.

Users

Health professional schools are, of course, the target user group. But provider institutions and individual health professionals will also want and need access to these materials, as will policy makers, researchers, and consumers.

Other Network Functions

Because the dissemination of education information is highly complex, it will be coordinated by an information service center that is part of the Education System. Medical schools will be able to purchase and use multimedia-based materials at several locations around the campus. But other users might not have access to a multimedia environment, or they may want only a subset of a learning module, and a more up-to-date one at that. Rather than have each user contact the national center directly, it is more efficient to have various versions of the learning modules available at regional service centers, or downlinked regularly to local service centers, for direct access by these other providers.

213

As is the case with the Guidelines System, the Education System outlined here meets the applicable framework criteria for a "good" health information system.

National Policy Formation Information System

Many health care policy-making groups have concerns about how to obtain adequate information and tools for good decision making. These groups include:

- Federal government bodies, such as the U.S. Congress and branches of the Public Health Service, including the Health Care Financing Administration and the National Institutes of Health
- National health care–related organizations, such as provider corporations, professional societies, and insurance companies
- Large special interest groups, such as pension funds and corporations that purchase health care for large groups of people: state, regional, and local governments; and researchers and educators

They all want answers to questions such as these:

What should the priorities be?

What is right or fair to do?

How should it be done?

When and where should it be done?

What is the best cost?

The information needed to answer these questions spans all aspects of health care, from determining the health needs of the population served to understanding the process of care delivery, including the amount and kinds of facilities and personnel needed, the outcomes, and the costs. It also includes census and geographic information. Moreover, as planners for the future, policy makers need this information over time in order to detect emerging trends.

Once these health care policy-making groups find that the information they need is already being collected (with every regard for confidentiality) at the grassroots level by provider institutions and public health and other government agencies at all levels, they will be able to capture the information for a hypothetical Policy System and then channel it as needed to the local, regional (or state), and national levels. Assuming that policy makers also recognize that, even more than just access to information, they need a sophisticated capability for managing and analyzing the information to make it useful to policy makers who are neither technically skilled nor medically trained, they will want computer-based tools that can perform these essential functions:

- Maintain and update the policy information database
- Prepare routine reports automatically
- Provide fast, easy access to subsets or combinations of the information in the database
- Perform statistical analyses
- Create models of aspects of the health care system that can be studied to improve understanding
- Conduct simulated policy decisions so that they can be tested on computer models rather than the American people

The assumption here is that collectively these groups will decide that even though the development will be long and arduous, it needs to be done with all due speed to avoid billions of dollars of future waste in the health care system. Further, they recognize that information technology can reduce their ongoing operating costs to a small fraction of what such costs might otherwise be. Their first step will then be to create the coordinating function.

National Center for Policy Information

The National Center for Policy Information, or the Policy Center, will formulate the framework for the National Policy Formation Information System. The network for this system, informally known as the Policy System, is shown in Figure 10.3. Because of the magnitude of the task, each metropolitan or comparable area will have an information service center to collect information in a privacy-protected manner from local providers. The assembled local information will be routed to a regional information service center where it will be combined with other such regionally based information as that supplied by provider corporations, insurance companies, and states. From there it will be routed to the national information service center at the Policy Center, where it will be combined with information from other regional centers and from such national databases as the Medicaid-Medicare and census databases.

At the local, regional, and national levels, all information collected to that point and all the processing tools developed by the Policy Center will be available for policy makers who need it at each level. Both standardized and customized analyses and reports will be made available.

Figure 10.3. Policy System Network.

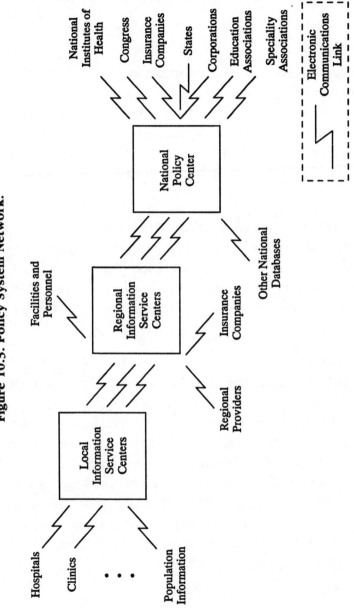

Suppliers

Providers who have the information about basic medical care in their patients' records will be the primary suppliers. Others will be the owners of numerous health care–related databases at all levels and, for example, the owners of the results of research such as surveys conducted especially for policy formation in specific areas.

Aggregation

The huge, never-ending task of virtually every aspect of aggregation will take place at the local (including provider), regional, and national levels. Each level will not only receive and process information but also analyze and format it in hundreds of different ways to meet the needs of diverse policy makers, researchers, and educators.

Brokering

The contractual agreements to acquire information and use it within the context of the Policy System will be formidable because different users will want different information in different forms. But this, of course, is the reason for the Policy System. Other important decisions to be made concern what information will be kept, for how long, and in what form. These challenges relating to health care will dwarf similar information system challenges faced by the Internal Revenue Service, the Social Security Administration, and the military.

Users

The founding user group has already been identified, but it is not an exclusive group. Regional planning groups, which by and large do not exist today, will be major users. A health care infrastructure, which we are assuming here has already been developed, will also be a big user, if not in fact the originator and owner of the Policy System.

Other Network Functions

Other functions will primarily involve dissemination, which will be carried out by the information service centers or their agents. These centers will be very complex, reflecting the diversity of perhaps thousands of requests each year.

Following are a few examples of policy formation in which the Policy System could play an important role in helping to make policy decisions more realistic.

The National Institutes of Health could develop a needs basis for setting research priorities.

The Health Care Financing Administration could use models and simulations to test proposed changes in Medicare reimbursement procedures before instituting them.

The Executive Branch could use health care system models to simulate health care payment mechanisms and then weed out unsatisfactory models before expensive and disruptive regional demonstration projects were funded.

Congress could use simulations to test the effects of Medicare spending cuts prior to enacting them into law.

The medical education establishment could assess the number and kind of health personnel that would be needed in ten years.

Regional planning groups could base their projections on sound demographic information.

Local governments could use the policy information to decide how public money should be used for health care programs.

All groups could use the databases over time to evaluate expeditiously and make adjustments in the effects of their policies on the health care system.

It is important to note that all these groups will use information from the same information stream, which will be generated and managed by the Policy System. Instead of having to make a special effort to collect evaluation information, these groups will find that information for evaluation is now just another by-product of the system.

As is true of the Guidelines System and the Education System, the Policy System described here meets the information framework criteria for a "good" health information system.

Beyond the Suggested Networks

Because each information system described above is national in scope, there is no need for duplicative development of guidelines, education programs, or policy databases by individual stakeholders or groups. Their suppliers in all three cases are similar in that all of them use the patient record or products of it and all of them use aspects of the medical knowledge base. Further, they use each other's products: the Guideline Background Databases, the new learning modules, and the policy databases. They all have the same geographic network links (provider-local-regional-national and/or the reverse). Thus even these few uses of the National Health Information System illustrate the economies it would be possible to make through avoidance of duplication of services and facilities.

The foregoing examples of possible national health care networks are neither inclusive nor exclusive. Many other possibilities and aspects could be explored within the context of each hypothetical network. For instance, in the Guidelines System it is unlikely that providers would want only guidelines; they would also want to have access to the Guideline Background Databases so that they could understand the rationale behind the guidelines. In the Education System, we would consider whether the guideline databases would constitute an adequate basis for reforming the medical school curriculum or whether some other portion of the medical knowledge base might be more suitable.

Some of the other aspects of the suggested specialized system networks will be discussed when we examine barriers to achieving the networks and the role of brokering in their development in Chapter Eleven. However, each example is already sufficient to show how the networking basics described in Chapter Nine come together to achieve a specific information function for specific health care system needs.

Other health care system needs that are ideal candidates

for specialized health information systems include the following:

A unified billing system

A quality-assurance system

Consumer health maintenance

A unified patient record

The process of medical education

Outcomes research

Primary care research

Outpatient services research

Chronic care services research

Several national health care–related information systems might at first appear to be specialized health systems, but they do not in fact fit our criteria. A brief look at two of these will help define more clearly just what kinds of systems are and are not subsystems of the NHIS.

The Medicare-Medicaid Information System (MMIS) was designed to meet management needs for an automated payment system within the Health Care Financing Administration. In general, systems with purely administrative functions would not be a part of the NHIS unless they impinged substantially on the processes of health care. The MMIS has done just that because its databases have been used extensively for health services research and they were used to develop DRGs as the basis for implementing the prospective payment system. Nevertheless, since its contribution is its databases, the MMIS would be considered primarily a supplier network to the NHIS rather than a specialized health care information system itself.

MEDLINE is the National Library of Medicine's information technology–based system of accessing the indexes of its holdings and finding and ordering materials of interest. This system, then, functions primarily as an information service center for aggregation and dissemination.

Each of the hypothetical networks described in this chapter has been presented as a fully developed and functional system, the development of which would require extensive resources and years of work. It is a characteristic of a good system that all its products (outputs) be goal directed and have value; such is the case with the systems (that is, the specialized subsystems of the NHIS) presented here. In each case, value would begin to be realized very early in the development process. To illustrate, the payoff from the Guidelines System begins as soon as the first guideline is disseminated, and the Education System has value from the time its first module is ready.

This is not an argument for incrementalism, however. The promised economies and synergies can be realized only when the goal is an NHIS with a complete set of interlocking, fully functional subsystems. But it does show that even when the NHIS or a specialized subsystem of it is only partially complete, it can begin to serve a useful purpose.

Chapter Eleven

Challenges to Developing a National System

The National Health Information System has been presented as an opportunity and a necessity for health care reform, but many tough issues surround its development. Among the issues facing advocates of an NHIS are those that directly affect our ability as a nation to *begin* its development. Three of these issues are discussed in this chapter:

- Barriers to initiating NHIS development
- The role of brokering in exposing and resolving more sensitive issues, both initially in network development and on an ongoing basis once the network is established
- Fundamental ownership and control of the NHIS

Barriers in Specific Systems

We begin by examining some of the major barriers common to the examples presented in Chapter Ten—and indeed to the other candidate systems as well.

Clinical Guidelines Information System

Barriers to development of the Guidelines System include those discussed below.

Networking technology. The nation's "information highway," which is the physical communications network on which the Guidelines System would be implemented, is discussed as a building block in Chapter Twelve. Today, the information highway—the backbone network—exists only in a rudimentary form, but the national development of a suitable communications network should keep pace with the remainder of the Guidelines System development. Even though the tasks of development and connection with the backbone network are well understood, much work remains, including making tremendous quantities of basic health care information machine readable so that it can be transmitted where it is needed for manipulation by computer programs.

Skilled personnel. The system developers and other technical people who would design, develop, and staff service centers at all levels are scarce.

Guideline Background Databases. The biggest challenge in implementing the Guidelines System is our lack of knowledge about how to create, represent, and manage the complex Guideline Background Databases. The inadequacy of the tools available to work effectively with complex databases is a technical barrier on which computer scientists are now working. But there is a health care system barrier as well: the lack of a well-established taxonomy for health care, which would be essential in this case.

Knowledge about disease processes and the effects of various treatments is not adequate either.

The biggest challenge is to organize the background information into a meaningful form. For example, if the primary index of the database were to be by name of publication, date, and author of a research finding, it would not be very helpful in explaining the rationale behind a guideline. More appropriate alternatives must be found to allow information from research articles to be combined more usefully.

Leadership. Within the health care system, the most immediate barrier to achieving the Guidelines System is the lack of agreements necessary to begin implementation. The greatest need is for stakeholder recognition of the importance of a Guidelines System and a commitment to develop it. The natural focus for such leadership would seem to be the professional specialty boards. While some guideline development is taking place today, it is being done in the absence of planning for the widespread and effective use of guidelines in clinical practice. The system of guideline creation, dissemination, and use could be imposed from outside by Congress or by insurance companies. But such a system would not be a "good" one, and it would cause further major compensatory dissonance in health care.

Education System

Barriers to implementing the Education System include those described below.

Networking technology. As is the case with the Guidelines System, networking technology is a barrier that should no longer exist by the time the information content, aggregation, and brokering functions are operational.

Skilled personnel. Computer-based health education specialists who could design the new modules and direct their development are scarce, as are the professionals who would maintain the materials and develop and staff the information service centers.

Materials design. The biggest barrier here is the unsuitability of the Guideline Background Databases for use as learning materials. Adapting them for use in education will be the task of the health education specialists. Although this development is a huge task, it can be accomplished by spreading the work over all the nation's health professional schools.

Faculty reorientation. Because faculty would be involved in developing the material, presumably they would develop an understanding of its importance and a commitment to its use.

Preexisting conditions. This information system is predicated on the existence of the Guideline Background Databases and on a preapproved curriculum redesign, neither of which exists yet and both of which would be very difficult to achieve.

Reward system. Presently, faculty involvement in developing learning materials is not generally rewarded by promotions, raises, or the granting of tenure—a situation that could and would change. Clinical students, too, would need a new reward system based on information management and utilization skills rather than on memorization of facts.

Medical education establishment. Today, medical schools are free to teach in whatever way they choose. The Association of American Medical Colleges, which is the medical school analog of the American Medical Association, can conduct studies and make recommendations, but it has no power of enforcement (*Educating Medical Students,* 1992). It is difficult to imagine where the system-wide leadership for the kinds of changes engendered by the Education Information System would come from. It is possible that financial pressures on medical schools (such as through their research budgets, student loans, or direct subsidies) would be used by Congress in an attempt to encourage change; again, compensatory dissonance would undoubtedly be the result.

Policy System

Barriers for the Policy System include those described below.

The physical network. The policy needs alone could strain the resources of the envisioned backbone network, but this is a technically surmountable problem.

Skilled personnel. The kinds of people needed do exist, but not in the quantities required.

Quality of data collection. Although rather ordinary kinds of information would be needed, the scope for error in information gathering and processing is extensive. Naturally, policy formation can only be as good as the information on which it is based.

Information compatibility. Linking the diverse databases needed to supplement the information collected directly from providers is both a technical and a medical problem. That is, databases developed at different times and places for different purposes may be incompatible not only in structure and format but also in such medical content areas as terminology, definitions, and relationships.

Accessibility of patient record. Much of the information needed for policy formation would be obtained as a by-product of an automated patient record, which does not yet exist. However, near-term developments sophisticated enough for the policy information system are likely.

Leadership. Policy makers do not yet appreciate how much better informed they could be if they implemented the Policy System. Nor do they understand that with sound planning and a long-term commitment such a system is entirely feasible.

Classes of Barriers

It is useful to group barriers to NHIS development into the three classes of explicit, emerging, and implicit barriers, since a different approach is needed to overcome the barriers in each class.

Explicit Barriers

Many of the barriers cited in the previous section are explicit: they are easily identified; they pose genuine challenges that we already know must be faced; and we know how they should be approached.

Technology-based barriers include the lack of a comprehensive communications network to which individuals and institutions can be linked; the incompatibility of the equipment (hardware) and computer programs (software) currently used by different suppliers, aggregators, and users; and the incompatibility of database structures, formats, and access methods.

Skilled personnel barriers include an inadequate number of medical informaticians who are specially trained in the application of computing in health care; the lack of socially oriented computer scientists needed to develop and implement the systems at all levels; and the as yet unidentified visionary scientists and scholars in health care who can guide developments.

Medical knowledge base barriers include the lack of common agreement on standards, terminology, and definitions for health information; an accepted taxonomy (hierarchy, relationships) for medical information; a concept of how the complexity of medical knowledge ought to be organized and presented for optimal effectiveness; and an orderly way of acquiring new knowledge and evaluating and integrating it with existing knowledge.

Product development barriers pose challenges to find new ways of looking at information so that new information products such as guidelines and learning materials can be conceptualized; to invent new tools in areas such as language analysis, text-handling methodologies, and research; and to research and develop adequate computer-human interfaces.

Leadership barriers pose special challenges that go beyond understanding problems and solutions or having the desire to act. The challenges include overcoming the political and social forces that mitigate for the status quo, especially of the existing health care culture.

Costs in general are not considered to be a barrier because the NHIS should be viewed as an investment rather than an expense. However, some aspects of costs are barriers. To the extent that overtech costs are unnecessary, they drain money from the system, money that could be used to plan and build the system's future. To the extent that profits from health care delivery are removed from the system (for instance, by shareholders), those funds are also not available for the system itself.

Emerging Barriers

Some barriers have not yet begun to exert their negative influence, but they deserve special attention because they will prove to be exceptionally thorny obstacles to a wholly satisfactory NHIS. They cut across several of the same arenas in which explicit barriers exist and all specialized areas within health care.

Computer-Human Interface. Computer use has been limited by health care workers' dissatisfaction with the computer keyboard and two-dimensional, black-and-white screen. Although this barrier is beginning to lower, in the future the complexity of the information relationships that need to be presented will require much more sophisticated interfaces. For instance, a patient record that is organized like an n-dimensional spreadsheet will require an interface that portrays at least three dimensions, thus extending current concepts of the use of information technology in health care.

Integration of the Patient Record and the Medical

Knowledge Base. With an NHIS, the patient record would be fully automated, the medical knowledge base usefully organized, and reliance on practice guidelines commonplace. The up-to-the-minute guidelines would be delivered to providers over the network, with background information available for each guideline on request. Physicians would probably study the patient record, make notes, and then either (a) scan the guidelines and select the appropriate set or (b) enter the patient's information into a guidelines program, which would then match the patient's problems to the appropriate guidelines and make suggestions.

However, providers would still be in a position of information overload. Therefore, the next natural development would be for the guidelines program to scan the patient record on command and offer its suggestions without the physician's having to reenter the information. This step is absolutely critical to acceptance of automated delivery of guidelines, and it implies that the guidelines program must be as much a part of a patient record system in hospitals and clinics as the drug interaction program or the lab results reporting program is today.

Type and Quality of Information. Even the vast storage capacity available through information technology could be overwhelmed by the collection or retention of unneeded information, information that is neither relevant nor timely. This problem applies equally to patient records and research findings.

Finally, if all relevant patient information is subject to use for research, then it must be of research quality. High-quality data collection (completeness, correctness, timeliness) must become second nature to all health care personnel. Errors in information must assume the importance of errors in treatment.

Implicit Barriers

Implicit barriers underlie every aspect of the NHIS.

Systems Analysis. The system needs a thorough assessment of its information needs and its options for meeting those needs.

Information Privacy. Privacy of patient, provider, and institutional information will continue to be an issue as long as certain medical conditions carry a social stigma or have financial consequences. These consequences might include failure to get/keep a job or insurance, failure to win a provider contract, or being liable in a malpractice suit.

Ownership of Information. The issue of ownership of information relates to whether the patient or some institution/body in the health care system owns patient information. At issue are *control* and *value.* As long as patient information is not used beyond its original purpose of communication with and between providers and as long as providers do not accept money for external use of the information in the record, ownership can continue to be a minor issue. However, when the information could be used to the detriment of the patient, say, in denying him or her insurance, or when it has monetary value, the issue will become critical.

If the information is used to the detriment of providers, then control becomes an issue. If information has monetary value, then the question becomes whether providers or patients or both should be paid.

Culture of the Health Care System. The system has a pattern of accommodating to change rather than being an agent of change—a role it must play in the development of the NHIS. Moreover, there is no doubt that information technology opens the door to change in organizational structure and the nature of work (Jarvinen, 1992; Parasuraman and others; 1992; Wagner, 1992). Fear is a barrier as long as information technology is unconfronted and its introduction not controlled for the benefit of both individuals and institutions. Only information technology–literate professionals who understand the power of the technology will be able to help define and shape the systems of the future to best meet their needs.

The health care computing industry does not have a great track record of service to the provider community. Early information systems did not live up to their promise, thus creating a credibility problem that has endured for decades between vendors and developers on the one hand and the health care community on the other. Even today, use of hospital systems for much more than administration and communication is limited, and use of systems in clinics is even more limited. Most providers have not really had the time and resources to consider what a positive contribution information technology could make to health care.

Special Interests/Conflict of Interest. Information flow in the health care system poses a real threat to many individuals and groups in health care. Those whose primary mission is not the same as that of the health care system are especially at risk because improved information flow could bring this fact to the attention of policy makers. Examples include companies whose primary mission is to bring profit to their shareholders, providers who take advantage of opportunities for overtech in their practices to increase their incomes, and providers whose standards for quality of care fall short of health care system standards. Such groups are expected to oppose increased reliance on information technology in the health care system.

Brokering Functions

This section focuses on expanded brokering functions that can help overcome the initial barriers to NHIS development described in the preceding section. First, we review *operational brokering* functions, then contrast them to *developmental brokering.*

Operational Brokering Functions

Brokering functions to be activated once agreements are made to develop and operate an NHIS include those governing the flow of information, such as routing, scheduling, determining conditions of use, pricing, and purging information. These particular functions are relatively straightforward. Other operational brokering functions such as compliance are more subtle in that they involve instilling trust and finding ways to ensure that trust is warranted. These functions constitute the *art of brokering* and involve such significant tasks as the following:

- Guaranteeing privacy and security of information
- Respecting ownership of information
- Guaranteeing quality of information
- Guaranteeing supplier protection from the inappropriate use of supplied information

Guaranteeing privacy includes preventing disclosure of individual physician names in the course of conducting institutional quality of care studies. It would also prevent disclosing patient identification on records used for, say, retrospective research studies.

The art of brokering would guarantee physical security such that, if the network were used for a consultation, patient information and the consultant's advice could be seen only by the two physicians involved or their designates.

The issue of who owns the basic information to be used in the NHIS has just begun to be debated. Whatever decision is made, the owner is not likely to have physical possession and control. It is therefore very important that the NHIS brokering component respects ownership in carrying out such functions as accounting and authorization for use.

Guaranteeing quality is an issue in preventing flawed research studies or erroneous patient record information from being used in guideline development, for instance. This is not to say that the NHIS would pass judgment on the value of specific studies or records; rather, its brokering function would ensure that mechanisms exist whereby such studies or errors in records were either prevented or detected and removed from consideration.

Guaranteeing supplier protection from liability for misuse of supplied information goes to the heart of the role of users in an NHIS environment. Having adequate information for decision making would not relieve the user from the responsibility to understand the information provided and make the ultimate intelligent decision. This pertains to all users, including physicians' use of guidelines, teachers' use of learning materials, and policy makers' use of databases and modeling programs.

Now let's look at a consultation scenario in which all these brokering functions play a role. Notice particularly that the art of brokering—instilling trust that the implicit guarantees are in place—is very much in evidence.

Dr. Peterson's patient Laurel Akins presents a puzzling array of neurological symptoms that defy categorization. He finds the therapeutic guidelines ambiguous in this case and decides to enlist the help of Dr. Shaw, a physician who is more experienced in this field. In response to Dr. Peterson's electronic mail note sent this morning, Dr. Shaw agrees to review the patient's records while she has lunch in her office.

Dr. Peterson authorizes Dr. Shaw's electronic access to Ms. Akins' records, and Dr. Shaw reviews them while munching a sandwich at 1:30 P.M. The multimedia information technology environment in her office enables her to review not only electronic pages of notes and test results at her terminal but also graphs, MRI images, and film clips from Ms. Akins' physical examinations.

Again using electronic mail, Dr. Shaw sends her analysis and recommendations to Dr. Peterson. In her note she explains the constellation of findings that led her to select the guideline she recommends. She also cites the portion of the Guideline Background Database that supports her reasoning so that Dr. Peterson can study it and comfortably reach the same decision.

Now let's examine the role played by the art of brokering in this example. Note that both the doctors and Ms. Akins believe that her record and the consultant's note are completely confidential because they understand that the NHIS is a secure network. Ms. Akins' privacy and ownership of her record are respected when the information service center (perhaps the computer facility in Dr. Peterson's clinic) verifies her wish to have relevant portions of her medical record released for this purpose. The only charge is a small service fee, which is added to her bill. Both doctors trust that the patient record is complete and accurate, and they believe that the guideline is correct and accurate in that it reflects the latest research findings; they are comfortable with relying on both information sources. However, what the two doctors decide should be done for the patient, on the basis of their study of the patient record and the guideline, is their responsibility (just as it is today). Ms. Akins trusts the two doctors; she believes that they have used the best possible information and are making the best possible decision. Thus in the electronic information age of the NHIS, as is the case today, it is necessary to build and sustain an environment where systemwide trust and individual responsibility work together. Such an environment is not automatic; it must be created and nurtured.

It is evident that the NHIS cannot function in the absence of these guarantees. This scenario highlights why a piecemeal commitment and specialized systems developed in isolation cannot succeed. The NHIS will not work if, for instance, only some provider records or only specialized portions of them are guaranteed for quality. Similarly, it will not work if only some portions of the network are secure, only some guidelines are verified, or patient or provider privacy and ownership are respected only part of the time. The commitment of all stakeholders is essential.

Developmental Brokering

Developmental brokering refers to brokering that attempts to overcome the barriers that prevent us from beginning the development of an NHIS. Without this type of brokering, about the only progress that can be made toward an NHIS is installation of the physical backbone network and prototyping (developing simplified examples of) specialized applications. Here is an ordered list of the barriers involved.

1. Ignorance
2. Fear
3. Lack of vision and leadership
4. Information incompatibility
5. Costs
6. Inadequate resources

Sample solutions for these barriers show how developmental brokering might work.

The best antidote to *ignorance* is education.
Health professionals and policy makers need a
vision of what an NHIS-supported health care
system will be so that they can create and take
advantage of opportunities to learn and contribute.
The developmental brokering function would be
to create that vision and the attendant learning
opportunities.

. For patients and providers alike, social and legal
reforms that destigmatize certain health information
could reduce the level of *fear.* That is, disclosure
of health information should not be cause in our
society for losing—or failing to get—a job, a
contract, or health insurance. For providers in
particular, a new attitude toward quality-assurance
procedures is needed. Review of therapeutic decisions, processes, and outcomes for purposes of
quality assurance should not be punitive; it should
be considered routine feedback that leads to education and changes in provider policies as necessary.
Fear of the workplace changes that will be possible
and likely in the information age can be met by a
sense of control over the future. Informed health
care professionals and other workers are in the best
position, collectively, to redefine and redesign their
own jobs. Informed, proactive health professionals
and policy makers who take charge of the design
and implementation of the NHIS have the best
chance for achieving that control and creating an
NHIS to their liking. Developmental brokering

would identify and work toward the legal and social reforms needed to protect patients and providers, and it would help empower health professionals and policy makers to design their own NHIS.

3. *The need for visionary leadership* is the primary reason that there is presently no health care infrastructure to create an NHIS. Tens of thousands of health care professionals know that a systemwide infrastructure, involving all stakeholders, is needed to plan for and create the health care system of the future. We need an infrastructure that represents not the stakeholders but the mission of the health care system in a way that no individual stakeholder group can. The capacity of health professionals for collective action to create that infrastructure is limited by the need for people of vision, accomplishment, and the power to persuade. The vision needed is one that would provide a context within which specific developments could be planned for and achieved. Developmental brokering would help identify and empower leaders, who would in turn empower educated, concerned health professionals who share their vision.

4. The NHIS's initial primary resource is a vast array of *incompatible information*. Patient-record databases, if they are automated at all, currently use different terminology, definitions, formats, and codes, and they vary widely in terms of the software that can access them. Other databases that are part of the medical knowledge base, such as

drug databases, are similarly incompatible. Creating compatibility requires general agreement to meet a commonly derived set of standards or criteria. The brokering function would work toward defining standards in both the technical and medical areas and obtaining agreement to use them.

5. As noted earlier, the *cost* of developing the NHIS should be considered an investment. Nevertheless, two aspects of costs should be noted. First, to obtain initial funding, the infrastructure would have to create a solid justification and plan for an NHIS. Second, costs for an NHIS would need to be controlled. The key element in controlling costs—in addition to good management practices such as planning and accountability—is the economies achieved through planned use of a common physical network and planned multiple uses of information collected once. Developmental brokering would facilitate planning, funding, and cost control for the NHIS.

6. The *resources* of skilled personnel and sophisticated technology, especially interface technology, will be needed. Developmental brokering would identify necessary resources and lay the groundwork for making them available by the time they are needed.

This section has shown that the brokering function is a very sophisticated one that is the lifeblood of the NHIS. Without it, the suppliers, aggregators, and users would be helpless. We have seen that brokering is much more than just information order taking and delivery; it begins with obtaining and coordinating a complex set of agreements, continues operationally by ensuring that information needs are met, and continuously evaluates its own performance.

Network Ownership and Control

Thus far we have conceptualized the NHIS by introducing the idea of specialized health information systems, which would actually be subsystems of the NHIS, to meet specific health care information needs. Then we showed how these systems should be treated as part of a whole—rather than as isolated systems—by examining the common barriers to their development and the brokering functions that would break down those barriers.

At the beginning of Chapter Ten, readers were invited to imagine that the health care system itself had initiated, developed, and now owns or controls these specialized subsystems and their networks. Those who did so will have reached this paramount conclusion: to reduce to manageable proportions the complexity and cost of each individual development, a health care system infrastructure needs to harness the information in all its patient records and its medical knowledge base and make it available uniformly throughout the system for multiple purposes.

Of course, the NHIS can be implemented at least in part without the leadership of the health care system infrastructure. In the absence of such leadership, it is just a matter of time until government agencies or groups from the for-profit sector begin negotiating directly with individual providers and groups for routine access to their patient records. If the resulting guidelines and education materials were developed by the government, for example, then we might expect that their use at some point would be mandated. If they were developed in the for-profit sector, no doubt they would be used to reduce the costs of the organization that developed them and perhaps be made available to other health care system users for a fee. These approaches would be in keeping with the systems principle of equifinality whereby in a good system there are several paths for reaching a goal.

Patient records, however, are the health care system's crown jewels, and they should be used in the best interests of the system as a whole. It would be a missed opportunity indeed if the health care system allowed others to profit from the development of its most fundamental resource. Of secondary concern is the potential for expensive and redundant private development of products based on the patient record and the medical knowledge base, an expense that the country can ill afford and that can be avoided.

It is appropriate that the health care system take the lead role in developing the NHIS because only the health care system has the brokering capability to break down the barriers that are hampering that initial commitment. Health care professionals alone cannot construct the NHIS; government and private businesses must play a role too. Commercial firms have a role in supplying hardware, software, communications, systems integration, and management and support personnel of all kinds. They would also take primary responsibility for aggregation and operational brokering functions. Governments have a role as catalysts, coordinators, and funders. They also offer an incentive to the health care system to take the lead role in NHIS development: they will develop the NHIS if the health care system doesn't!

PART THREE

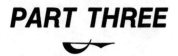

Making Transformation
a Reality

Chapter Twelve

Indicators of Progress

The National Health Information System is the information technology–based mechanism for meeting the information flow needs of the health care system as defined in its information framework. Although the NHIS does not exist today, the idea of the need for one is not new. A trend toward developing such a system was already apparent in the late 1970s, and it was discussed formally on several occasions in the early 1980s (Duncan, 1980; Austin, 1981; Kaple, 1981; Klainer, 1981). In fact, in 1981 a congressional hearing was held on the need for a national coordinated health information system (*A Coordinated Health Information System,* 1981; Duncan, 1981). More recently, a number of public and private groups have called for a national information highway for health care, including most notably the Institute of Medicine's Committee on Improving the Patient Record (Dick and Steen, 1991, p. 51).

This chapter integrates the individual ideas of the NHIS, first by showing the characteristics and flow of information for the NHIS, and then by describing the hypothetical experiences of an information-liberated hospital that extensively uses a fully operational NHIS. Next, the chapter examines work going on in several arenas that could serve as building blocks of the NHIS. A distinction is made between projects that are truly building blocks and other projects that apply information technology in health care. Finally, this chapter considers the role of the interprofessional discipline of medical informatics, the community that is best prepared to lead NHIS development.

The National Health Information System

As explained earlier, the initial objectives of the information framework are to develop and facilitate the use of these key resources: an accessible patient record, the medical knowledge base, and outcomes research results. It is clear from the many examples cited that the NHIS would be ideally suited to meeting these objectives because it would be designed and implemented to have the following characteristics:

- It would recognize health-related information as its most valuable commodity.
- It would facilitate and ensure systemwide information flow.
- The commitment to information flow would come from all levels in the system.
- Information would routinely be of high quality and reliability.
- The information needed would be appropriately available, regardless of its source or destination.

- Relevant new information would be readily integrated with old.
- Disparate information from multiple sources could be integrated.
- The system would have adequate safeguards to ensure security and protect privacy and ownership of information.

Note that this list of characteristics does not include information technology because the point of the NHIS is not to create a huge computer network but to meet complex and extensive information flow needs by using computing and communications. Therefore, our focus continues to be on information-based requirements rather than on the technology. It is sufficient to say that the national network on which the NHIS would be implemented would be as unobtrusive to health professionals as the national telephone network, despite all its many routes, technologies, and carriers.

The backbone network, or information highway, would connect national centers to regional centers and to each other, as shown in Figure 12.1. The health care system would share the information highway at the national and regional levels with a host of other information services such as cable television and applications such as education and basic science research—just as is the case with the telephone network and the interstate highway system. Individual providers and other local suppliers/users would access the information highway either directly or through local information service centers. Connecting to the NHIS would not be a problem because almost any personal or

Figure 12.1. National Health Information System.

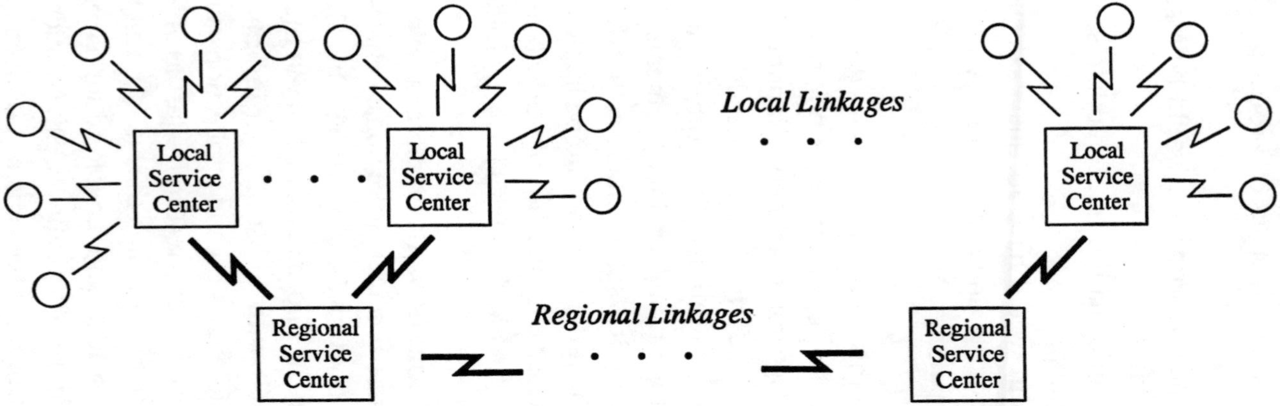

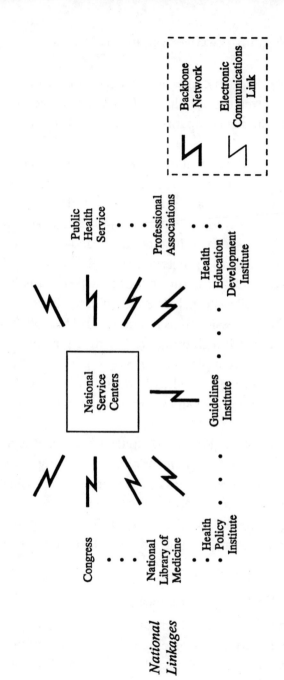

institutional computer can easily be made capable of connection. (However, the usefulness of such simple interfaces is severely limited in comparison to the complexity of the tasks.)

To show how the overall network would function from the perspective of an individual health professional, let's examine how health care professionals and others associated with a medium-sized teaching hospital—called Roberts Hospital—located in a medium-sized city, would hypothetically relate to the network in the future. Although this example is set in the future, nothing about it is far-fetched. In fact, all the capabilities noted have either been recognized by professionals as important and feasible (for example, database integration), are in active planning or development (for example, guidelines, computer-based patient record), and/or have already been implemented in health care or other disciplines (for example, national networks).

An institution like Roberts Hospital would, as it is today, be using information technology for many intra-institutional purposes, such as ordering, results reporting, and using a drug interaction database. These we will take for granted as we look more closely at the new capabilities that would be available to Roberts Hospital through the NHIS.

New Local Networking Capabilities

Extra-institutional demand for information from the patient record has triggered development of local networks with regional and national links. Health professionals and consumers can access most information through computers in their offices or homes as well as from computers in the Roberts Hospital library, offices, and study rooms or at the bedside. The range and diversity of information available are undaunting to today's users because they have already given their own systems a great deal of information about their needs and preferences. A series of menus eases the remaining choice selection.

Early in the development of the NHIS, hospital-based automated patient record systems became much more sophisticated. Using only the hospital's own capabilities, professionals are additionally now able to conduct personal research projects using the patient and other hospital databases, such as comparing their own utilization of hospital goods and services with utilization for similar diagnoses in the hospital as a whole.

Using only the local network, professionals can communicate from the hospital with their homes, offices, or other local institutions on the network. In fact, a centralized community health record system is being developed at the local information service center for the convenience of all community providers and consumers.

Services for Roberts Hospital's Medical Staff

A range of new information services is available to help physicians manage their work. Many decision aids are available to physicians, including reminders, databases, simple rules, guidelines, and expert systems.

Clinical guidelines that advise the physician in diagnosis, treatment planning, and continuing care have been developed for most patient problems. The guidelines, and the Guideline Background Databases, were developed at centers throughout the country, as described in Chapter Ten, and are validated, maintained, and distributed by the national Guidelines Center. This center distributes new and updated guidelines regularly through a national information service center to regional centers. The regional centers have standing orders from each provider/institution as to which guidelines it needs and in what format and schedule.

In addition to the guidelines themselves, computer programs generally known as *expert systems* are available to guide the physician as desired through the Guideline Background Databases—and other related databases especially developed for this purpose—to understand the scientific basis and research that contributed to formulation of a particular guideline. At Roberts Hospital the guidelines, expert systems, and other advisory programs, such as drug interaction databases and internal cost/benefit studies, are made available on demand or automatically.

When a doctor reviews a patient record, the advisory programs may review it as well, or the physician may enter information himself. Advice on how to proceed is then returned to the physician. If the physician asks for an in-depth justification of a recommendation, the query may be routed to the appropriate Guideline Background Database and back, through the regional or national information service center, but the delay is so short as to be insignificant.

Without reference to a particular patient record, physicians may use the NHIS to *investigate* any topic in the guidelines, the Guideline Background Databases, other medical knowledge databases, or even original research articles. They do not need to know the name or location of the databases because the regional information service center will interact with them to help find and select any databases and material relating to the specified topic(s).

Personal research is commonplace, as physicians can quickly and easily conduct studies on questions that have caught their interest. They may use the local patient record database to look for correlations with information from a local environmental database, for example. They may also have noticed and verified correlations in their patients' records that are not mentioned in the guidelines—thus painlessly contributing to the medical knowledge base. In fact, physicians' informal research studies will have contributed to the refinement of guidelines more rapidly and completely than would have been possible if studies had been commissioned to close the gaps in the guidelines. The Guidelines Center maintains electronic mailboxes just for such contributions. Physicians can use the NHIS to forward findings on the spot and become valued members of the guidelines development team.

Because of the accessibility of the patient record and the ubiquity of multimedia workstations, interinstitutional *grand rounds* can be conducted over the network with other groups throughout the country. Physicians who contract to participate can share records and even "converse" interactively over the network during grand rounds. The multimedia workstations make it possible to show film clips and other images over the network as well. Similarly, *consultations* can be obtained from distant colleagues.

Multimedia materials are developed for *continuing medical education* at virtually every medical center in the country, and accredited materials are made available over the NHIS. The local service center maintains the list and finds and routes a copy for the provider to use whenever and wherever she may be.

Physicians can also *review the learning materials* developed for health professional students at the National Health Educational Development Center to brush up on basic science, clinical, or other related skills. Subsets of these materials are maintained at Roberts Hospital because it is a teaching hospital; others may be obtained from the national Education Center via the information service centers. The materials may be studied at the provider's convenience.

Physicians can register on a variety of automated local or national *bulletin boards* to obtain information of interest and post their own information at will. Some bulletin boards physicians can select to scan routinely are notification of local, regional, and national meetings or seminars in a subspecialty; bulletins from drug companies; public health notices; new product announcements; research news flashes; state and national legislation; and minutes of specialty-board business meetings.

Opportunities for Other Health Professionals

Nurses, technicians, social workers, and other health professionals have the same access that they have always had to patient records, and they have the same access that physicians have to the guidelines and all other databases.

They have the same opportunities for research, review of learning materials, access to bulletin boards, and access to continuing education materials accredited by their professional societies. In addition, they use electronic mail to take advantage of the rich opportunities to exchange information and ideas with colleagues in similar positions around the country.

Opportunities for Roberts Hospital's Administrators

Hospital administrators have found a gold mine in the NHIS. Patient and provider information has become a valuable commodity in a health care system that for decades suffered from deep ignorance about its own characteristics and workings. The hospital works hard to maintain the quality, completeness, and diversity of its information to maximize the demand for it.

When Roberts Hospital's information is requested for *research studies* or the development of learning materials, for instance, the hospital earns a royalty over and above the minimum standard fees paid for routine information.

Because the patient record is automated, *billing and cost accounting* for services is completely automatic. Payers have access to the same guidelines as physicians, so delays due to disagreement over appropriate treatment have been greatly reduced. Information needed for assessment of the hospital's quality of care, accreditation, and other reviews and reports is also prepared automatically.

Because Roberts's administration is deeply involved in *regional planning,* administrators use the in-house videoconferencing facilities extensively to "meet" over the NHIS with regional planning groups and national policy makers. In preparation for these meetings, administrators conduct research by using demographic, facilities, and personnel databases, which they access from regional information service centers over the network.

The administrators also use the videoconferencing facilities to meet with *health plan negotiators.* Their research is elaborate, involving the use of cost and outcome databases, as well as demographic, facilities, and personnel databases and such ancillary information as relevant legislation and regulations. All this information is available over the NHIS, either from the regional planning centers or the national Policy Center.

Administrators have network access to current and historical materials catalogued by the Policy Center, including *local, state, and national legislation and regulations* and their current status, amendments offered, and prospects. They can obtain individual *research articles,* abstracts, or summaries of research in selected areas, analogous to clinical guidelines. Administrators can use local and national *news and information services* such as CompuServe, Prodigy, or Dow Jones News. They can *review learning materials and use continuing education programs* for credit. Moreover, administrators have access to all kinds of *bulletin boards,* which alert them to current contents, potential problems such as product liability, and conferences and workshops of interest. Of special interest are postings of people seeking hospital jobs and jobs that are available.

Opportunitites for Students

Roberts Hospital has both undergraduate students and residents on its clinical services. Because the standard medical school learning modules are generally available over the NHIS, *undergraduate students* from the regional medical school who rotate through Roberts Hospital can study clinical material as well at the hospital as on campus. They are at Roberts to learn how to interact with patients. Working with individual physicians, they experience clinical decision making firsthand by learning how to create an effective patient record, use the guidelines and other databases, and review research studies. They also participate in or conduct their own clinical research studies by using the local patient record database, participate in grand rounds, and use the bulletin boards.

Residents use the NHIS in the same way that staff physicians do. However, their focus is on studying the guidelines, using the background databases, and reviewing original research materials. They make extensive use of computer simulations of (real) patients to practice their decision-making skills and pinpoint areas needing more study. Because their careers will require lifelong learning and contributing to the profession, they also use the local patient database and even Roberts Hospital's patients to conduct extensive clinical research studies.

Consumer Services

As has been the case for years, and whether or not they are patients, consumers are free to use programs and information derived from the medical knowledge base, including guidelines, research articles, and learning materials. Of course, they do not have access to any patient records except their own, either individually or in the aggregate. Groups all over the country have developed health-related educational materials especially for patients and other consumers. All these materials can be accessed at one of Roberts Hospital's libraries or in the consumer's home or office. Programs that discuss and describe home care are also available for review in patients' rooms prior to discharge.

We have now seen the entire spectrum of typical information flow in the NHIS from the point of view of a single provider institution: how information goes from providers to the regional and national levels for research, development, and policy; and how basic patient information and developed information products and databases are combined, recombined, and refined for use in patient care and in further research. All these things are possible only when all stakeholders are connected and contributing.

Building Blocks and Related Developments

People who know something about computers and health care might say that most of the applications just described are already being done, and without the NHIS. This is not the case. While it is true that there are information technology applications throughout the present health care system, almost none have had any impact on the nature and quality of care on a systemwide basis except as noted in Chapter Eight. Even the guideline, education, and policy systems described in Chapter Ten are simply health care applications, not true building blocks. However, we are not exactly at the beginning, for much work of value has been done.

Prototypes

Although limited in scope and not directly applicable to the NHIS, some applications have shown the potential for information technology. Much of this seminal work is described in *A History of Medical Informatics* (Blum and Duncan, 1990). Key projects that have laboriously but surely created paradigm shifts in the health care system include the following:

• The first successful hospital information system developed at El Camino Hospital in Mountain View, California, in the late 1960s. The system has demonstrably reduced errors and costs (*Demonstration,* 1977).

• The Problem-Oriented Medical Record, developed by Dr. Lawrence L. Weed in the 1960s. Weed's landmark article about patient records, which appeared originally in 1968 in the *New England Journal of Medicine,* was reprinted twenty-five years later and is even more relevant today. He showed us that the patient record could indeed be organized and that advice could be incorporated into a patient record system. He also espoused the notion that a patient should have a single continuous, coherent record. In support of that notion, in 1968 Weed told us:

263

It has been said that preoccupation with the
medical record and the computer leads to ne-
glect of the "humanitarian" side and the "art"
of medical practice. The most humanitarian thing
a physician can do is to precisely know what he
is doing, and make the patient as comfortable as
he can in the face of problems that he cannot yet
solve. There have been major humanitarian and
sociologic failings in medicine, but almost all of
them can be attributed to our poor behavior as
scientists as we have dealt with problems out of
context and ignored data relevant to good medical care [Weed, (1968) 1993].

- Disease-specific registries, such as a tumor registry,
which were first implemented on punch cards but have
been automated since the days of the first computers.
These registries have demonstrated the value of trolling
the patient record for clues to further research.

Building Blocks in Progress

Still other projects seem to be genuine building blocks for
the NHIS for several reasons. They support the needs of
the health care system so that it can meet its mission, and
they cut across and would benefit all arenas of information
flow in health care. Further, each project gives attention
to the critical steps of developmental brokering, the biggest developmental need today. That is, project resources
are devoted to educating key players, raising their com-

fort level, enlisting support, and reaching agreements. Following are some examples.

The Computer-Based Patient Record Institute (CPRI) is an outgrowth of the Institute of Medicine Committee on Improving the Patient Record's recommendations (Dick and Steen, 1991). The institute was founded in 1992 by a number of stakeholder groups to foster the development and implementation of computer-based records. It is working in these key areas: standards, education, CPR infrastructure, systems evaluation, and facilitation of adoption (*Computer-Based Patient Record,* 1993). CPRI represents an enormous conceptual breakthrough. Almost overnight the computer-based patient record went from something only a few off-beat visionaries really believed should and could happen to an establishment-endorsed probability. It is the first good example of health care system stakeholders' collaboration.

CPRI is a building block because, like the NHIS, it presents the computer-based patient record as an important information resource for uses throughout the health care system. It supports the mission of the health care system in every way. CPRI also has a program of outreach, education, and encouragement aimed at health professionals to enlist their support.

The upsurge of interest in *hospital quality improvement* is a building block because the NHIS will not work unless reliable information is the norm. Of particular interest are projects that use the methods of total quality improvement (Berwick, Godfrey, and Roessner, 1990).

Medical informatics research is a discipline that in part seeks to understand the nature of medical knowledge and make it more relevant and useful in the practice of medicine. As such, it studies and develops tools and techniques for creating decision aids for clinicians. Medical informatics research is a building block because it is developing the fundamental ideas and technology that are essential for bringing clinical guidelines and expert systems into the NHIS. Further, its work is applicable throughout the health care system because these same ideas and technologies will bring medical knowledge to students and consumers as well as to providers.

Internet is the forerunner of the information highway, a project that enjoys considerable political and commercial support. Internet is the existing backbone network developed originally by the U.S. Department of Defense to connect defense research facilities throughout the world. Currently, individuals in research-related corporations, academic institutions, facilities, and organizations around the world use the network for many purposes, and its estimated seventeen million users send several million electronic mail messages every day.

The capabilities of Internet, beyond the original Department of Defense intentions, have not been marketed, and it offers no user services (although its member subnetworks may do so). The network was simply made available and the response has been phenomenal. Internet is a building block because its mission of facilitating electronic information flow for health care (among other things) is entirely congruent with the mission of health care system and essential for the NHIS. Further, it has helped to break down personal barriers to electronic communication by overcoming prejudice, ignorance, and fear.

Internet's capacity is inadequate for future needs, and plans are under way in both the public and private sectors to fund and develop the high-capacity, high-speed physical network the NHIS needs. Schools at all levels and medical and research facilities will be high-priority users.

NHIS-Supportive Developments

Many interesting developments and uses of information technology offer experience and ideas to health professionals regardless of whether or not they are actual building blocks for the NHIS. Several key projects are described in this section. Some are in the medical field, others are in technical areas, and a few pertain to other developments in our society. For more information about the use and potential of information technology in health care, the reader is referred to "Information Resources" at the back of this book.

Patient Record Systems. Here are some record systems that have enjoyed at least local success and garnered national attention.

- Technicon Medical Information System (TMIS), El Camino Hospital
- Computer Stored Ambulatory Record (COSTAR), Massachusetts General Hospital
- Health Evaluation through Logical Processing (HELP), Latter-Day Saints Hospital

- Regenstrief Medical Record System (RMRS), Wishard Memorial Hospital
- The Medical Record (TMR), Duke University Medical Center

The Personal Health Record. Underlying the intriguing work on the Lifespan Personal Health Record (Williams, Imrey, and Williams, 1991) is the notion that there are many advantages to having each individual maintain his or her own patient record, a concept that is central to the rationale for creating an NHIS. If we are to reduce the use of acute-care medicine to an acceptable level, we must have tools such as this to help individuals accept responsibility for their own health. The proposed record would probably use an electronic accessible memory card, and it would include information provided by the consumer as well as information provided by health care providers. It would also be "expert" enough to monitor the card contents and offer some guidance to its holder.

Outcomes Research and Guidelines Development. Guidelines are being given a boost in many quarters. Several professional societies, or specialty boards, are developing guidelines specific to their specialties. The Rand Corporation has contributed significant pioneering work in clinical guidelines development. The Federal Agency for Health Care Policy and Research's (AHCPR's) Medical Treatment Effectiveness Program (MEDTEP) has four elements: "medical effectiveness research, development of databases for such research, development of clinical guidelines, and the dissemination of research findings and clinical guidelines" (Salive, Mayfield, and Weissman, 1990, pp. 697–698). The MEDTEP work is based on two assumptions: that "variations in clinical practice are associated with differences in outcomes and resource use" and that "inappropriate practice patterns can be changed if relevant scientific evidence is effectively disseminated to health care providers and patients" (Raskin and Maklan, 1991, p. 164).

Standards. The matter of standards applies both to health care and to information technology. In health care there is a need for standards for terminology, definitions, taxonomy, and format. In technology there is a need for data-exchange standards to achieve hardware, software, and database compatibility and information security. Progress is being made on many of these fronts, especially those pertaining to the computer-based patient record (*Automated Medical Records,* 1993).

The National Library of Medicine (NLM) has been sponsoring development of the Unified Medical Language System (UMLS), the goal for which is to map the terminologies used in several different medical databases into a common language. The American Society for Testing and Materials (ASTM) and the American National Standards Institute (ANSI) are each developing vocabulary and technical standards. Health Level Seven (HL7) and the Institute of Electrical and Electronics Engineers are also working on technical standards.

Research Methodology. The massive clinical research needed for definitive guidelines development—an iterative process that will take decades—needs new, less cumbersome, and less time- and resource-consuming ways of obtaining and using information. For instance, it is possible that the AHCPR's ambitious Patient Outcomes Research Teams (PORTs) will not be able to carry out their research missions cost-effectively without new approaches, including new research concepts, tools, and techniques.

Recent reports on progress in new research approaches come from the U.S. General Accounting Office on new research designs and from the AHCPR on linking databases (*Feasibility of Linking,* 1991) and research methodologies (Fowler, 1989; Grady and Schwartz, 1992; Sechrest, Perrin, and Bunker, 1990).

Emerging Technology. Two key aspects of technology, the backbone network and the development of standards, have already been mentioned. Although much work remains to be done for the NHIS on both aspects, current technology is more than adequate for the state of development of the other aspects of the NHIS, such as automating the patient record and creating an accessible medical knowledge base. It will be an exciting day when the health care system can complain that it is being held back by the technology.

Computer-human interaction (CHI) is a singular case where better technology would help even today. Because most medical information still has to be entered into a computer by a human being, we need better devices for doing this. Health care professionals and others want to enter and retrieve data wherever they are, such as at the bedside or walking around, and they need the power of a computer "workstation" to do these things. Before too long, clinicians should be able to take a powerful wireless computer terminal out of their pocket and use it wherever they are (Bria, 1993).

Users who do not need such portable computing will soon find exciting new options as well. The learning environment, for instance, will include multimedia workstations that incorporate (1) communications capabilities for phone, fax, and telecommunications; (2) video, stereo, photos and diagrams, and computer-generated images retrievable from compact discs or remote locations; (3) the intellect-extending power of computing itself; and (4) imaginative interfaces for interaction with computer programs. All of these will be elements of computer-based learning modules.

A natural way for consumers to get the information they need and to maintain their health records and advice programs will be through the emerging technology of interactive television (ITV). People will be able to order up personalized health care and medical information through ITV just as easily as they can shop or access information services. However, even these interface tools will not be adequate for the full-blown NHIS. Emerging technologies such as neural nets, fuzzy logic, and virtual reality will then come into play.

Related Developments. The NLM's Integrated Academic Information Management System (IAIMS) program helps medical centers create campuswide network integration between electronic information resources and information users. The Duke University Medical Center model illustrates the complexity and utility of such a network (Stead and others, 1993). Much of what can be learned from

271

IAIMS projects is directly applicable to the development of the local aspects of the NHIS.

Information services such as Prodigy, MCIMail, CompuServe, and the Dow Jones News Service are teaching us a great deal about how to provide a wide variety of information sources in a useful way, and electronic publishing is on the horizon as well. The future relationship of these nonhealth industries to health care is explored in Chapter Thirteen.

Medical Informatics. The new discipline medical informatics must be included in this discussion because it is from the ranks of its practitioners, medical informaticians, that NHIS developers are most likely to come. One aspect of the discipline, that of medical informatics research, has already been discussed as a building block of the NHIS. The other major aspect is that of developing applications of information technology in health care. The discipline as a whole is content rich and complex. Most medical informaticians have a doctoral-level degree. Those who wish to become medical informaticians must study one or more aspects of health care, such as clinical medicine; computer science, or at least how to use the technology; and concepts specific to the integration of health care and the technology. About thirty programs exist to train medical informaticians. Many of these programs are supported by the NLM. As a result, the nature of the training programs, and therefore the nature of the discipline, reflects the NLM vision ("A Vision of the Future," 1986).

Medical informatics has been in existence at least informally since the late 1950s. The first formal doctoral-level model curriculum was developed under the auspices of the Education Board of the Association for Computing Machinery (Duncan and others, 1981). Because the group that developed the curriculum recognized even then that the discipline was too complex and extensive to be encompassed by all graduates, it devised four specialties and acknowledged that even more specialization might be required over time. This has certainly been the case.

While medical informaticians are working on many important problems, not enough of them are working on problems that are key to developing the information framework and NHIS. Although information technology is used extensively in health care, that use is not necessarily leading us in the direction of an NHIS—the direction that is essential if the health care system is to move beyond the current crises and avoid future ones.

Chapter Thirteen

Visioning the Transformed System

Earlier scenarios of an information-liberated health care system were built directly upon the impact of removing the information logjam from the existing health care system. Those scenarios represent the minimum NHIS development necessary to alleviate the current crises in health care and avoid the dissonant future scenarios presented in Chapter Three.

In contrast, this chapter presents an integrated set of scenarios of what *could evolve* in an information-liberated health care system. These scenarios go beyond the immediate impact of the technology discussed thus far to reflect a community that has transformed itself into a vibrant, mission-oriented system. Although everyone may not consider them desirable because they would require that the health care system continue to put aside stakeholder differences, they do illustrate how a mature system could evolve, grow, and function to the benefit of all legitimate stakeholders. They reflect the natural result of a systems approach to change.

The Status of Information

In the mature health care system, information liberation through the NHIS will be recognized as the transforming agent that has freed the system from the tyranny of too much—and too little—information. The NHIS will have freed the system from expending its resources on administrative detail, low-level clinical decision making, and routine transmission of information. It will have offered options to increase the quality, quantity, and pace of research and development in clinical care, self-care, policy formation, and education. In short, it will have liberated the health care system to focus on *extending the art and science of health and medicine and achieving universal health.*

In that climate, the view of information will be totally different from today's view, in which hiding personal information has primacy and the need for an integrated knowledge base is not yet widely recognized. In the mature health care system, information will be treated as a valued commodity to be shared. Although protection of privacy will always be essential, medical conditions will be destigmatized and viewed merely as individual variations. The NHIS will be organized as a utility that offers information, communication, and the derivative information services of brokering and aggregation on which all health professionals, students, consumers, and policy makers may draw.

Health Professional Education

The transformation scenarios begin with physician education. In comparison with today's health professionals, future providers will have the much richer educational experiences made possible by the NHIS and the more open attitudes that they will need to function effectively in the mature system.

As part of the early reform movement, information technology will at last be used to assess accurately the quality of care delivered by different types of providers, including medical students and residents. As a result, consumers will no longer be willing to participate in the system of allowing unqualified medical students and residents to make patient care decisions. By then it will be widely recognized that students really do need to learn a set of clinical skills in medical school instead of trying to memorize patterns for specific patient problems and that they can learn these skills by using the NHIS *before* they present themselves as physicians to their patients.

Among the key skills that will be needed are (1) skills in caring for patients, (2) skills in clinical decision making, (3) skills in using information resources for lifelong learning, and (4) skills in conducting research. Computer-based simulations that use clinical decision-making tools in diagnosis, treatment planning, and prognosis will be commonplace, allowing the gradual separation of early training in decision making from training in patient care, to the great benefit of both kinds of training.

Learning Patient Care

The present-day student-patient encounter is unsatisfactory for both parties. Unfortunately, from the time of the student's first clerkship, one of the first things he or she must learn in clinical medicine today is how to be comfortable with not knowing exactly what to do but doing something anyway. This sets up a barrier between the patient and would-be physician whereby the latter must gain the trust of the patient in spite of the knowledge that the relationship with the patient is not entirely honest.

In the mature health care system, the student's encounters with patients will be based directly on the type and level of training the student has had. Students will not present themselves as physicians. Instead, they will experience the health care system with the patient, and from the patient's point of view: they will become the advocates of the patients under their individual care and thus be able to focus on being of genuine help to them.

In both primary care and hospital or medical center settings, students will be assigned a rich caseload of patients for the duration of a rotation. Their task will be to come to a complete understanding of their own patients' problems and the decisions being made on behalf of their patients. Students' mentors will be all of those patients' physicians, whose time will have been freed so that they can be responsive to the students' need to gain a full picture of each patient. In the course of these activities, students—both generalist and specialist candidates—will be evaluated on such objectives as these:

- Learning to think of patients holistically
- Learning the skills of listening, understanding, and developing a genuine advocacy relationship with patients and their families

277

- Learning how to get information for their patients, and teaching their patients how to get information
- Learning and carrying out for their patients routine ancillary health care functions from such disciplines as nursing, patient education, physical therapy, laboratory, dietetics, and transport
- Learning about and participating in physicals exams, history taking, and other patient interviews (but not presenting themselves as physicians)
- Learning how to perform, and performing, community service through such avenues as preparing and teaching wellness programs or helping in clinics

Although patient-care students will not at any time present themselves as diagnosticians, they will work closely with their physician-mentors to understand completely and justify the decision made for each patient.

Learning Clinical Decision Making

Students will begin their training in clinical decision making (CDM) in parallel with their training in patient care. To learn CDM skills, students will draw from a rich set of computer-simulated "patients" based on real patient records and use all the tools (guidelines, decision aids, databases) available to clinicians for diagnosis, treatment planning, follow-up, and prognosis in caring for these "patients." The simulations will, of course, be supplemented by texts, didactic assignments, seminars and rounds, and original research to give these future physicians every opportunity to acquire and practice the skills of lifelong learning.

278

The simulation programs and information resources will be available at all health care facilities, thus regionalizing medical education by freeing early clinical students to participate in a variety of health settings, including those in geographically underserved areas. By the same process, residents will be able and required to study CDM and work with patients in outpatient as well as inpatient settings. The diversity and accessibility of new clinical settings, combined with the simulation programs, will allow students to gain experience with a much wider variety of problems than is possible today.

Learning records will be maintained by the computer system to monitor which simulations the students have used successfully. After the students have "practiced" on a full range of simulations in a given clinical area, they will be tested with further simulations to be sure that they have learned how to use all the relevant information resources. When the students demonstrate mastery, they will then be eligible to become primary physicians for patients in that clinical area. This same process of training, evaluation, and certification for patient care will continue throughout their residency.

Integrating Patient Care and CDM

Patient-care students will already have had experience in integrating patient care and CDM as they developed a holistic view of their patients. Thus, when they become qualified through their studies in CDM to see patients as physicians, they will be ready. As students and residents, they will only be assigned as primary physicians for patients in the clinical areas in which they are fully qualified. It will be an easy matter in either an undergraduate or residency program for a computer program to scan the patient record and students' learning records to identiify which students are qualified to be assigned to a patient. Their CDM skills, combined with their patient-care skills, will have prepared them in a most humane and complete way to treat patients effectively.

Acquiring Research Skills

Clinical research skills will be needed not only for lifelong learning but also for learning how to make lifelong professional contributions to health care. From their first rotations, medical students will be assigned clinical research problems that require the use of the patient database and information from the medical knowledge base. At first, they will repeat exemplar studies to gain experience in using the full set of information resources, with evaluation by the computer system. Subsequent studies will progress with increasing degrees of sophistication, originality, and utility.

Faculty Rewards

The faculty reward system will reflect the new attitudes and capabilities generated by information liberation. Because of the NHIS, clinical research will be much easier to conduct, and electronic publishing will all but eliminate the laborious preparation of research papers. Instead, results (for which faculty will be paid) will be forwarded directly to the appropriate Guidelines Development Center for evaluation and integration with existing knowledge.

In addition to their research contributions, faculty members will receive rewards based on their development and maintenance of learning modules and on the time they spend mentoring. Even though faculty will be expected to spend a significant amount of time with students, the time will be spent in teaching patient care, managing, and mentoring, while the simulation programs convey the basic CDM skills.

Educating Other Health Professionals

The need for a transformation that separates training in patient care from training in clinical decision making is particularly strong in physician education. Patient care is already integrated more appropriately in other health professions. However, the shift to extensive use of computer-based learning materials and the focus on lifelong learning and research will occur in all health professional education.

The Clinician's Office

Many facets of the future clinician's office have already been presented. The ideas that follow focus on transforming aspects of information technology use.

Clinical Gaming and Continuing Medical Education

Working with simulated patients is fun. Health professionals of all varieties will enjoy pitting their skills against complex patient problems that, while derived from real patient records, now exist only through a computer program. These programs will give health professionals the opportunity to explore new options and learn from others' approaches to the same problems. Caring for simulated patients will serve as the basis for contests, and several related cases will be used for rounds. Moreover, health professionals will even construct their own simulations to share with their colleagues or contribute (for a fee) to the pool of learning materials.

Simulations and other clinical decision aids will, of course, also have a serious purpose in the clinician's office. They will offer a means of routinely monitoring clinical skills. Based on the clinician's performance with these programs, continuing education may be recommended; this in itself may take the form of a simulation.

The Integrated Office

Completely automated case management will be routine in the office of the future. Computerized patient records will be monitored routinely, according to the clinician's specifications, and quality assessment data, bills, reminders for appointments, test results, and recommendations for preventive care or educational programs will be routinely and automatically sent to office personnel, external agencies, or patients as appropriate. For the clinician's convenience, not only the patient record but the medical knowledge base materials and aids and continuing medical education programs will be fully automated and integrated. These conveniences will free clinicians and their staffs to concentrate on the patient as they learned to do in their professional schools.

The Clinician-Patient Relationship

The clinician-patient relationship will be transformed into a true partnership. Although the clinician may have advice and therapy to offer the patient, it will be recognized that the patient holds the keys to the success of the partnership. First, patients, or clients, have it in their power to remain well and thus eliminate the need to see the clinician. They also have it in their power to participate in preventive care. If they do see the clinician, they have information the clinician needs in order to decide what must be done. The power of compliance with therapy is theirs as well.

Electronic communication will make it possible for offices to send reminders, education material, test results, bills, and new or requested information directly to their patients' home computers. Conversely, patients can send payment, follow-up information, or home test results to the clinician's office. This latter capability will greatly facilitate chronic care. But the options for using electronic mail will be the most transforming. With electronic mail, patients and office personnel, including clinicians, will be able to chat interactively and at their convenience about patient symptoms, appointments, or questions.

The Empowered Consumer

Information technology will make possible the transformation that finally empowers consumers to take responsibility for their own health and their use of the health care system. Four key elements are involved here: (1) the personal health record, (2) communication with providers as discussed above, (3) information resources, and (4) changing social attitudes toward health.

Each consumer will maintain a Personal Health Record, probably kept next to his or her driver's license. The record will contain not only the consumer's complete medical record, including hospital records, but also a health history summary and lifestyle information that is pertinent to health. When the consumer sees a doctor, she or he will present the record for automatic updating at the office or hospital. Using a home computer, the consumer will update her or his own record with information on diet, exercise, family medical history, and life events. At the same time, instructions already in the record will advise the consumer of any problems with the information being entered or remind the consumer of the need for a preventive test or an appointment. The consumer has the option of sharing any or all of the record with different providers.

The consumer's primary information asset will be interactive television, often attached to the home computer. The medical knowledge base, already in public libraries today but almost impossible to use, will have been formatted for the use of nonhealth professionals through interactive television. The programs will function like a menu of information services from which the consumer may use a remote control or home computer to choose information as diverse as first-aid advice, advice about whether symptoms warrant a message to the clinician, detailed information about the cause and course of a specific disease, or side effects of certain drugs. Information may be presented in text, graphics, animation, or videos—or in entirely new media.

The Transformed Patient Record

Much has been written about the need to automate the medical record and the many derivative uses it will have in the future. However, even when records are automated, for some patients, the information will be so complex that it will still be difficult for clinical personnel or researchers to grasp fully the contents and their implications. There will be simply too much information to be kept in mind at once. Many variables will need to be examined from different points of view, correlated with other variables and events over time, and presented simultaneously in an intelligible way. When it becomes possible to display the record in this manner, clinicians will be further liberated to unleash their creativity on behalf of patients.

Virtual reality is an emerging technology that may be able to crack the complexity barrier. Virtual reality systems construct an artificial three-dimensional world within which the user, wearing special goggles, perceives himself to be, and within which he seems to move around and interact with the environment. Although virtual reality is used primarily for arcade gaming today, some serious uses are beginning to emerge. Researchers at Carnegie Mellon University have used the techniques to develop a virtual car showroom within which visitors can "see," "feel," and "drive" a new automobile and to reconstruct the interior of a real Egyptian temple (Zengerle, 1993).

Analogously, a vibrant artificial world full of shapes, colors, sounds, textures, and movement will someday be constructed, based on the patient record. The clinician of the future will browse through and interact with this "virtual record"; in fact, several geographically separated people at once will enter the virtual record for consultations or learning simply by donning the goggles or other interface devices. They will also be able to test the effects of alternative therapies in the virtual world before using them on the real patient.

Clinical Research

The concepts of research-as-by-product, clinician-as-research-partner, and formal electronic publishing will be significant in the mature health care system.

Individual Physicians' Studies

During the period of early exponential refinement of the medical knowledge base and guidelines, developers will come to realize that, thanks to information technology, it will no longer be necessary to combine patients into arbitrary groupings for determining therapy. It will instead be possible to identify millions of different clinical patterns and then tailor therapy almost for the individual patient. To create these patterns for use in guidelines, individual physicians will be encouraged to conduct clinical research routinely in their practices. The quantity and utility of their research will determine the fees they will receive.

Group Studies

Standardized patient records, high information quality, and electronic communication will make it possible to conduct sophisticated research studies at community facilities. Specialized multifacility regional research networks will flourish, marketing their findings to developers of the medical knowledge base, especially for guidelines development.

Collegial Research

The Human Genome Project has been cited as an example of collegial research, research in which researchers throughout the world who have common interests can share analytic tools and information. This practice will become routine, spurring the pace of research because researchers in very narrow clinical areas will be able to communicate quickly and interactively. Collegial research will become possible after the formalization of electronic publishing, which will provide mechanisms for recording where ideas first originated on the network and who contributed to them.

Libraries and Publishing

Today the medical knowledge base, including library holdings, are a by-product of publications for individuals. Tomorrow the individual's use of information will be a by-product of the medical knowledge base. Clinicians will no longer need to read raw research findings, which are not really valuable to individuals until they are integrated with existing knowledge.

Publications will still be archived, but libraries will understand that they are in the information business, not just the business of archiving publications. They will understand that clinicians need integrated information rather than raw information and that it is no longer necessary for each individual physician to find, study, and integrate the same information. Working collaboratively with developers of guidelines and clinical decision aids, mature libraries will provide access to a full range of supporting information tools of value to clinicians, including the scientific rationale for each recommendation. These tools will already have integrated the latest research findings.

It will also no longer be necessary for years to pass before clinicians, researchers, and students can have practical access to research results. Several developments will make this possible.

- Data quality will improve.
- Research tools will become more sophisticated.
- Research skills will be more widespread.
- A number of new formats, including electronic submission, will be acceptable.
- Review criteria will shift to include review of the genesis of ideas as well as the findings.

The pace of research will be much quicker, and the cycle from idea to study to review to certification of the research to clinician will be much shorter. Formal electronic publishing, whereby credit is given for being the first to register ideas and findings electronically, provides a powerful incentive to speed research out of the laboratory and into practice.

Successful publishers, like libraries, will realize that they are in the information business rather than just the book and journal business. They will take responsibility for maintaining the guidelines and their accompanying background databases, developing interfaces, and providing access to clinicians, researchers, students, and consumers. A major source of publishers' revenue will be the fees for access.

Health Care Policy

Information technology–based tools for health policy will help introduce order and normalcy into the system. Artificial constructs that could lead to compensatory dissonance will no longer be possible. Therefore, stakeholders will no longer need to protect their legitimate functions from encroachment by other stakeholders or outside agents; cooperation and collaboration will be the norms.

Innovation in health care delivery will be greatly facilitated by the NHIS. Complete computer-based models of the health care system and its stakeholders and arenas, including models of their structure, functions, and resources, will abound. Proposed policy changes will routinely be tested on the models before being implemented in the real system.

Planning to ensure universal access to care through equitable and adequate distribution of resources will be the rule, as will careful attention to quality and cost of care.

Specialty and geographic distribution will be capacity controlled with financial incentives, and a National Health Service for education and care in underserved clinical and geographic areas will thrive.

New Role Definitions

With the NHIS, the kinds of health professionals needed in the future will not be exactly the same as before. More options will be available for people who would prefer a community-based profession rather than a science and research-based one.

Physicians

In the transformed health care system, all physicians will practice patient-centered health care, as taught in the medical schools of the future, but they will also be scientists. As the medical knowledge base expands and information resources become more sophisticated, the intellectual demands on physicians will increase accordingly. Their training as problem-solving scientists who can navigate complex information resources will be so intensive that their primary function will be to care for patients who have special needs for those problem-solving and caring skills. All physicians will be specialists because our society will not be able to afford to have such highly trained professionals delivering care that does not require their special skills.

Community Providers

Primary care will be delivered by a kind of health professional that does not even exist today—perhaps a "community provider"—and will not be the equivalent of today's family-practice specialist. The emergence of this new professional will result from a natural transformation of the system toward a cost-effective way of improving access and keeping people healthy and out of the acute-care system.

The new professionals will have the same general training that physicians do, except for a residency; instead, they will have a community-oriented internship that will lead to such responsibilities as prenatal care, well baby and child care, chronic care, preventive care, postinstitutional care, routine physicals, ordinary medical problems, patient and wellness education, community outreach, and front-line gatekeeping for the specialist system. Community providers will accomplish their training in five or six years of postsecondary school study. To assist them in their work, they will have access to the full range of automated tools, including case management systems and guidelines.

These new providers will initially come from the ranks of such health professionals as today's nurses, physician's assistants, physical therapists, social workers, and emergency medical technicians. Later, as transitional training materials are developed, unemployed professionals from all walks of life will be retrained for the role. Ultimately, this will become a very attractive career of choice for those who want to care for patients directly without becoming scientists.

Other Health Professionals

While current professions will not disappear, they may be different; certainly new kinds of professionals will be needed. The need will be greatest for professionals who can manage information and for community-based professionals.

The Necessary Nurses. What nurses do is so central to patient care that it is likely that medical and community provider students will carry out many of today's nursing functions in both hospitals and outpatient settings as part of their patient-care training. Nurses will have many options in the future, just as they do today. For example, they may continue to play the role they do now, teach patient care to a broader range of health professional students, or act as administrators, medical information specialists, or community providers.

Information Specialists. New professionals known as information specialists, will have a clinical background so that they will be able to work constructively with clinical information. They may choose to develop clinical databases and programs for the NHIS. Or they may choose to implement programs in user environments and teach their use. Or they may choose to work directly with information access on behalf of other health professionals. For instance, an information specialist may help a clinical team navigate a virtual patient record or test all the options in a new CDM program.

Community Educators. The mission of community educators will be to work with community providers in instilling the concepts of wellness, including prevention, public health, and use of information resources, throughout the community. They will develop wellness curricula and learning materials for public and private schools at all levels. They will also develop and carry out community outreach programs and offer special programs and support to community groups.

Home-Based Caregivers. Home-based caregivers will work with community providers to support homebound chronically ill or postinstitutionalized patients. This support will include education, monitoring, and care.

Consumers. As consumers learn more about wellness and how to use the health care system, they too will become a part of the health professional equation. They will make important health care decisions for themselves, decisions that today are being made for them or not being made at all.

Medicine as Science

Perhaps the most exciting transformation possible for health care is an intellectual one. The process of creating the Guideline Background Databases will spark new interest in the science of medicine as a whole. This new interest will go beyond the curative or problem-solving aspects to embrace a complete understanding of underlying healthy and pathologic body mechanisms and the effects of attempts to alter them. New emphasis on the individual will become the norm as professionals learn that no two people have the same "medical makeup" and therefore should not be treated in exactly the same way.

New information will suggest new holistic approaches to understanding disease processes, incorporating systems theory, chaos theory (Ditto and Pecora, 1993), and mind-body relationships. The new knowledge will begin to clarify the relationship of human beings to the planet and the universe. In fact, studies in medicine will contribute new clues about the workings of the universe, which are mimicked in all its elements, including humans. At last, medicine will join the family of sciences.

Transformation Summary

The foregoing integrated scenarios reveal aspects of a health care system that has used information liberation to meet contemporary challenges and then transformed itself. The centerpiece of the future system is the community provider, who will bring about universal access by extending health care and education into individual community units. The system of community providers can be achieved at a cost far less than that of trying to move highly trained physicians into practice situations where their skills are not fully utilized. Physicians will be free to work wholly within the acute-care system, where their skills are most needed. The health care picture is completed by the empowered consumer.

Also in place in these scenarios is the supporting infrastructure, consisting of the transformed educational system, research system, libraries, information flow, supporting personnel, and policy formation.

Much has been left unsaid, as it should be. The principle of equifinality tells us that in a healthy system there is more than one path to a goal. Some of the questions about where responsibility lies for choosing and embarking on a path will be discussed in the next and final chapter.

Chapter Fourteen

Beginning the
Process of Reform

The health care system has lost touch with its mission, and its stakeholders function in isolation, each pursuing its own goals. Time after time, the system has turned its back on opportunities to provide leadership in situations where medically trained leaders were essential. Its failure to develop a functioning infrastructure for problem solving goes hand in hand with its failure to lead, and the existing information logjam is the inevitable result.

Deepening Dissonance

As the foregoing forces continue to operate in the system, the resulting compensatory dissonance has disturbing implications for the future unless the health care system or the federal government recognizes the threat and acts decisively. Major emerging trends and ideas in the system are, in fact, serious compensatory dissonances that will further destabilize the system. While the intent behind them is good, they are powerful new forces being introduced outside the context of an overall strategy for reform. Primary among these are:

- The trend toward megacorporations of health care providers
- The attempt to reduce the federal deficit through cost savings in health care
- The notion of creating a higher proportion of primary physicians by reducing the number of new specialist physicians

These and other dissonances combine to threaten the system in at least these three areas:

- Quality of care
- Removal of resources from the system
- Failure of preventive medicine and wellness concepts

Quality of Care

A dramatically increasing interest in quality of care and the use of guidelines is evident throughout the health care system. At its heart is the untested belief that improved quality in the system will reduce waste and lower costs. Let's examine where this belief is taking the system.

- In provider settings where a commitment to quality improvement has been made, the focus is on improving institutional performance on such parameters as immunization levels, length of stay, or claims turnaround time. Working toward institutional-level performance goals is only peripherally a patient-centered activity, and it does not improve clinical decision making. In fact, widespread adoption of institutional performance improvement as a cost-saving tool diverts attention and resources from the much more important patient-centered problems of access and overuse, underuse, and misuse of health care technologies. Institutional performance improvement is a classic example of stakeholders attempting to solve a problem they can identify and solve rather than cooperatively seeking solutions to the problems that most need solving. When one-time savings have been taken, the cost spiral will recommence.

• Reducing clinicians' use of medical technologies can reduce costs, so large providers and groups will use their own information systems to generate guidelines for clinicians. When these take the form of quotas, incentives, and protocols for use that resemble rationing, they are not generally patient centered and must be considered contrary to the goals of the system.

• There is a danger that providers' institutions will require physicians to use institutional outcomes as guidance in clinical decision making. This is especially likely in situations where technology has not been evaluated sufficiently otherwise. Several researchers have warned against using outcomes at the expense of a focus on the scientific basis of disease processes, diagnosis, and treatment (Cotten, 1993; Eddy and Billings, 1988; Grimes, 1993; Wennberg, 1988). Approaches that do not use the full gamut of available information resources to develop guidelines may have a worse impact on patient care than no guidelines at all. Further, the tangle of different guidelines throughout the system will exacerbate provider and geographic variability.

- Some providers may possess sufficient sophistication and information resources to develop sound guidelines of genuine value to clinical decision making. They may even be able to develop enough of these guidelines to have a positive impact on their overall quality of care and costs. Unfortunately, the emerging mega-provider groups are preparing for a competitive health care environment, so each group will need to develop its own clinical guidelines, an enormous and unnecessary duplication that will drain the limited resources of the system.

- The AHCPR is engaged in the development of clinical guidelines for use nationally. Unfortunately, the resources of the AHCPR are miniscule in comparison to what it needs if it is to generate a critical mass of guidelines in, say, the next ten years. As long as powerful provider groups prefer to develop their own guidelines to improve their competitive position, AHCPR may be unable to command the resources it needs.

Removal of Resources
Many entrepreneurs believe that they can meet the federal containment goal and still generate a rewarding profit in health care ventures. This will be true in the short term.

As multiprovider corporations convert to managed care, they should be able to wring sufficient one-time savings out of the system to accomplish both goals for a few years. When the cost spiral starts up again, however, they will be faced with the goal-directed choice of cutting profits or the compensatory dissonance of cutting services. Meanwhile, because the conversion to managed care by itself is capable of doing little more than generating one-time savings, precious dollars will have been drained from the system with little to show in return.

The Failure of Preventive Medicine and Wellness

Current trends will not soon lead to comprehensive, effective use of preventive medicine or to improved health in the general population. Here's why.

• Because preventive medicine is thought to reduce system utilization, each provider group will devote resources to determining which preventive services are most effective in doing so. Over a period of several years, most preventive services will not be found to be cost effective and will be adopted only selectively, even though they may have great potential value to the consumers who receive them. For instance, a woman under fifty may want the security of having a regular mammogram, even though statistically the chance that a woman in her risk group has breast cancer is so low that it is cheaper for her provider to treat the occasional advanced cancer than to screen the entire group regularly. While it is unlikely that preventive services would be reduced to levels that would endanger

299

public health, this is no consolation to the patient who is denied the service and becomes ill with a preventable medical problem.

• The preventive service of health education and behavior modification will not be adopted at a level that can be shown to reduce system costs. Not enough is known about how to achieve success in entire populations groups, and experimentation would take years. To the extent that work will be done in this area, once again each provider group will develop its own materials and approaches to health education to maintain its competitive position. With the emerging focus on more exciting developments such as quality improvement, this area will get little more attention than lip service.

• There is general agreement that more primary care is needed, both to improve access to underserved groups and to refocus the system on keeping people healthy so that they will not need as much acute care. But contemporary systemwide models for primary care are not satisfactory, and research on new models is limited (Franks, Nutting, and Clancy, 1993). It is not known, for instance, whether "better" primary care can reduce costs and how such care should be delivered (Clinton, 1993). Although the AHCPR supports research in this area, years will pass before answers emerge. Meanwhile, the system is being re-engineered in the absence of good information about how to do it.

- Shifting the proportion of primary care providers by providing incentives to medical students to go into primary care will harm the system in both the short and the long run. First, our medical schools do not teach many key skills needed by primary care physicians. Second, as medical technology and the clinical decision-making process become more complex, we will need more, better-trained specialists and medical researchers, not fewer. Finally, as long as this approach holds out the false hope of a solution to the primary care shortage, resources will not be forthcoming to explore seriously other, more productive approaches, such as creating a new profession of primary care providers.

Reform or Change?

The driving force behind all the deepening dissonances is the pressure to make health care a less costly share of the federal deficit. The health care system must respond by controlling costs or face further government involvement in stakeholder affairs. The only mechanisms it has are those of its individual providers and suppliers, so that is where the cost-cutting work falls. Those individuals must respond; there is no one else to do so. Because they cannot respond appropriately, their responses will create further dissonance in the system within five or ten years. This is not reform.

Reform, including cost containment, will be achieved only when we find approaches that do not betray the mission of health care; we will only discover these approaches when we consider the entirety of the system. That is, we must consider not only the organizational aspects of health care but also its social context, its sociology, and most of all the clinical functions that are at the heart of the system and constitute its reason for being. The presumption is not valid that clinical practice can be disregarded in the reform debate because its scientific basis is well established.

Our failure to achieve as a nation the health care system we want has been our failure to understand the underlying causes of health care's problems. The failure of our health care system has been to leave the problem solving to those who do not understand. Change, not reform, is the product of this process.

The Path to Reform

Ongoing organizational and administrative changes at the institutional and multi-institutional level are already under way. No doubt sensible changes at the national level will soon follow, leading to improved access and uniform procedures for cost and quality accountability. The pressure cooker of unresolved issues will then center on getting the right kinds of providers where they are needed and on ensuring high-quality clinical decision making. To achieve this as a nation, we need to do the following:

- Move to a three-tiered system of care consisting of specialist physicians, a new and separate profession of primary care providers, and health associates who deliver noninstitutional services

- Reform provider education at all levels to meet the needs of the three groups of caregivers
- Establish enforceable mechanisms for allocating resources (people, facilities, and research monies)
- Commit resources commensurate with the scope of the problem to developing, disseminating, and enforcing systemwide guidelines and other clinical decision-making aids
- Commit adequate resources to systemwide research on the delivery of primary care and the maintenance of good health in the population
- Commit adequate resources to developing the National Health Information System, which must underpin all reforms

We are indeed fortunate to be living in an era where information technology is available because, while information technology cannot reform the system, health care cannot be reformed without it. The envisioned NHIS would support any kind of future health care system; the flow of information needed for decision making is independent of the use to which it is put. It is no coincidence, however, that the steps proposed above are the first steps toward the transformed health care system described in Chapter Thirteen.

To evolve gracefully to such a system, we need an *overarching strategy* within which *planned* experimentation with modes of delivery, *coordinated* guidelines development, and *efficacious* incremental changes can occur as they become feasible and affordable. How these reforms can be accomplished is problematic in the absence of a health care infrastructure because stakeholder cooperative agreement on goals and methods is essential.

Opportunities for Leadership

We now consider which communities and groups from inside and outside the health care system might lead the effort.

The Health Care System Establishment

On the practical, emotional, and intellectual levels, health care stakeholder groups and individuals know that their system does not work. They sense that the system is falling farther and farther behind in coping with cost containment, with decreased access, and with the information explosion. Further, they sense that the individual motivations they follow are not really right for society as a whole and for solving these problems in particular. As individuals, however, they do not regard the options for national change as being *their* options.

These individual attitudes are reflected in the attitudes of the institutions that represent the stakeholders of health care as well. Their official policy statements and recommendations for reform tend to resemble stakeholder holding actions against an impending doom rather than challenging, practical alternatives for the future of health care. Nevertheless, change is coming, and it will be imposed from outside the system if the system does not change itself. The only recourse for stakeholders is to redirect their commitment and resources toward working together to fulfill the mission of health care. While all stakeholder groups and individuals need to consider how they can make a difference, some groups would seem to have a greater responsibility than others by virtue of the position they have carved for themselves in the hierarchy of health care. These will be explored in more detail.

The Physician Community's Role. Health care system stakeholders seem surprisingly willing to allow the federal government to take the lead in most aspects of health care policy. The single exception is the unsurprising unwillingness of the physician professional and trade associations to relinquish the principle of physicians' personal professional autonomy. However, physicians will have no choice but to relinquish it unless they themselves act to make the necessary changes. The reason is very simple: physician decisions generate about 75 percent of all health care costs (Ginsberg, 1992), so cost containment would not be possible without involving physician decisions. In fact, the federal government has already made preliminary cost-cutting incursions into the physician's realm with DRGs and the RBRVS, and we have seen how destabilizing they can be.

The next incursion from outside has already begun: the control of guidelines. These can be a useful tool for physicians if they are developed, integrated, disseminated, and maintained appropriately—a tremendous task. Let's consider the options for control of the development and enforcement of guidelines.

- Under a single-payer system, the federal government will sponsor the development of guidelines and enforce their use by making them the basis for reimbursement. The physicians will be at financial risk for nonconforming clinical decisions.

- Under managed care, each provider group, such as an HMO or integrated health care organization, will create its own guidelines, which may or may not be directed more toward cost containment than toward quality of care. Each provider corporation will have different guidelines, and only physicians who agree to use them will be able to continue to participate.

- Under fee-for-service, third-party payers will each develop their own guidelines, and each will have different guidelines. These will be applied when the physician seeks reimbursement, putting the physician at financial risk that a claim will be denied.

- Under any malpractice reform, arbitrators or juries will use the guidelines offered by their expert witnesses. No doubt there will be as many different sets of guidelines as there are experts.

All these options would use diverse guidelines in punitive ways and primarily after the fact. While some credible groups are developing specific guidelines for use on a national basis, the pace today is so slow and uncoordinated that one or more of these scenarios is all but inevitable.

The best option is for the physician community to take responsibility for the development of guidelines that can be used under any payment mechanism or delivery system, thus relieving the perceived need for *post hoc* punitive guidelines. Physician leadership needs to begin by forming a cooperative and comprehensive policy group to plan, identify resources, seek support, and expedite coordinated guidelines development.

The physician community is in the best position to lead health care reform in several other arenas as sell. The community:

- Is uniquely qualified to understand what the health care system needs to do differently and explain this to the American people. Physician association policy statements should reflect a vision not of what is best for their members but of what is best for achieving the system's mission.
- Needs to take the lead in creating the cooperative environment of a health care infrastructure within which leaders of vision can plan for the future health care system.
- Must recognize the need for different kinds of clinicians if universal access to the appropriate levels of care are to be achieved.
- Needs to take the lead in formulating and implementing more appropriate medical education for all types of providers.
- Needs to address the information logjam directly by supporting development of the computer-based patient record, adopting computer-based case management, and working to achieve the NHIS.

These are all essential elements of effective development and deployment of guidelines.

The Health Care Community's Role. The ability of the health care community to lead and its continuing commitment to improving the system are evidenced in part by the community's initiative in establishing the national Computer-Based Patient Record Institute and the initiative shown by hospitals in moving toward integrated provider organizations. With the physician community, or as an alternative if necessary, the stakeholders of the greater health care community could jointly take national leadership in planning for the mission-oriented health care system of tomorrow and communicating with Congress and the American people about what needs to be done to achieve it: creating the essential health care infrastructure, initiating health education reforms, initiating primary care research, and establishing and credentialing much needed new practitioner groups.

The Federal Government

Reform leadership from within the health care system seems so desirable that the best approach would probably be for federal policy makers to facilitate their leadership while giving the health care community, say, five years to show five years' worth of progress toward cost containment, wider access, and quality improvement. Specific indicators of progress might involve meeting targets in guideline sponsorship and adoption, clinician distribution, refocused medical education, and activities promoting wellness. If the health care community is unwilling or unable to act at the national level, then clearly the federal government must take the lead in creating a reasoned, coordinated approach to reform that takes into account all aspects of the system.

The National Library of Medicine and Medical Informatics

Two other national communities are dedicated to understanding medical information and facilitating information flow and utilization in the health care system: the National Library of Medicine and the discipline of medical informatics. Both are working on important problems in these areas, and to a much greater extent than any other group. Further, they both have a long involvement with information technology. In 1966 the NLM first began its MEDLINE, which today gives individuals electronic access to the NLM's primary indexes. Medical informatics is even more integrated with information technology because it sprang directly out of the new computer industry in the early 1960s.

Both forces have the potential to lead the health care system toward the NHIS. Their credentials and the appropriateness of their leadership is clear. In fact, associates of both groups would tell you that information liberation is essential and inevitable and that what they do is directly related to the NHIS as described in this book.

Unfortunately, however, the operative world for both groups today falls far short of what is needed for the NHIS because their operative world is much smaller than the reality of health care. The vision of each is circumscribed by what it, as an individual institution or discipline, can do. Neither appears to see itself as a catalyst for the much larger effort that is needed. Let's take a closer look.

The National Library of Medicine. Despite its extensive commitment to and support of the use of information technology in health care information flow, the NLM appears to be falling farther and farther behind the curve of what can and must be achieved. The problem is one of scope and scale. In planning its agenda, it seems as though the NLM may not realize the magnitude of the information problems facing the health care system and the scope of the role it needs to play. It is almost as if the NLM is working at the molecular level of medical information when what is really needed today is a *vision* of the information-liberated health care system that would provide a *context* for the NLM's leadership in fulfilling that vision. The NLM should leverage its assets and prestige until it reaches the front of the information-liberation parade. Let's see how this can be done.

The NLM of today gives the impression of being an archival institution that is developing information technology–based tools to make its information more accessible and useful to health care professionals. The NLM that is actually needed would have as its primary mission the adequate flow of medical knowledge within the health care system to all who need it in fulfillment of the system's mission. The operative word is *adequate*. With this new mission in mind, the NLM could take the following steps:

- Take stock of itself and recognize that its solutions are falling behind the scope and scale of the information flow problems in health care today
- Acknowledge that those problems cannot be addressed by current approaches to the dissemination of medical knowledge
- Reconceptualize the nature of the medical knowledge base, not—as it is today—as the diverse, clinically less than useful collection of research findings organized by publication title, date, and author; rather, view it as a valuable, if incomplete, information resource that must be reorganized, integrated, formatted, and delivered to all people who need it and where and when they need it
- Recognize the urgency of the need for the reconceptualized medical knowledge base and the need for collaborative action to achieve it
- Identify, educate, and enlist the support and resources of other groups who should share that mission, from the health care system, government, and other public and private arenas such as the publishing industry
- Lead a collaborative effort to develop and implement an action plan for achieving the reconceptualized medical knowledge base
- Recognize the systemwide information context of the medical knowledge base (the information framework) and leverage its own talents and resources to build the rest of the information infrastructure as well

The totality of these steps would create a substantive base for the National Health Information System.

Medical Informatics. Medical informatics (MI) as a discipline originally encompassed virtually any use of computing in health care. As information technology has become more sophisticated, MI has over the years become increasing narrow; it is focused now in two primary areas, clinical decision making and clinical information system applications. Although its present work is important and necessary for the NHIS, as is the case with the NLM, there is first a question of scale and scope. In terms of scale, the work being done today is not nearly enough; the discipline is falling farther and farther behind what can and must be done. The pace is too slow, and there is little sense of the urgency of the problems. In terms of scope, many essential concerns are scarcely being addressed. Consider, for instance, the many barriers and brokering functions identified in Chapter Eleven.

When one considers the problems of the health care system, it is apparent that MI is developing solutions to problems that have been outpaced and outclassed by the information trends that have led to the current crises. Increasingly, the context for MI projects is to use information technology to work on some interesting problems. It almost seems as if MI is preparing to merchandise a technology rather than build a discipline or science. A *science* would be based on discovery of the world as it really is (Shannon, 1983), a context that seems to be missing in MI. The *context* for MI needs to be defined as what information technology can do to solve urgent health care problems (Duncan, 1992). That is, MI needs to work toward *transformation* instead of applications. MI leaders need to recognize the complexity of the task presented here as the NHIS and use a systems approach to embrace and accomplish the work that needs to be done.

The work of MI, like that of the NLM, appears to have a molecular orientation that does not take into account the contemporary health care system (Duncan, 1988). The computer-based patient record offers an example of the difference between the current *molecular approach* and the proposed *systems approach*.

- In molecular terms, the patient record is an inefficient document, and information technology could improve it. Many new and better things could be done in health care if the patient information were available electronically.

- In systems terms, clinicians' lack of good information about clinical options (the information logjam) is raising costs systemwide and jeopardizing quality of care. Therefore, the health care system needs to reconceptualize the medical knowledge base to make it more complete, accessible, and useful to clinicians. A reasonable approach would be to develop and deliver integrated clinical guidelines based on what we know. But we really do not have adequate outcome information to develop the critical mass of guidelines that would have an impact on the systemwide problems of cost and quality. If patient records contained high-quality information and could be made massively available electronically to dozens of outcomes research teams, we might actually be able to develop guidelines that

313

would have an impact in, say, ten years. However, that would be possible only if the patient records were available on a large scale within the first two of those ten years.

This scenario provides a context for seeking development of the computer-based patient record as a matter of the highest priority and urgency. Notice that the scenario is based on an *urgent system need* rather than on the availability of a molecular-scale problem and a convenient technology.

There are no other similar disciplinary communities that can take the leadership role in applying information technology to urgent health care system problems while leaving MI to continue its present, limited approach. Since information technology in the form of the NHIS is the key element in moving the system out of crisis, MI professionals have an obligation as professionals to lead.

Conclusions

Sadly, the health care system will continue to be buffeted by pressures from within and without unless and until leaders emerge who understand the forces at work and are ready and able to act. The National Health Information System holds the key to unlocking the complexities of clinical practice, building a more effective system of care, and freeing the consumer to stay well. Information liberation within the health care system is not a new idea; it is simply an idea that has never captured the attention of the system as a whole. Perhaps now, however, it is an idea whose time has come.

Information Resources

Associations

American Healthcare Information Management
Association
919 North Michigan Ave.
Chicago, Ill. 60611-1683

American Medical Informatics Association
4915 St. Elmo Ave., Suite 302
Bethesda, Md. 20814

Association for Health Services Research
1350 Connecticut Ave. N.W., Suite 1100
Washington, D.C. 20036

Healthcare Information and Management Systems
Society
230 East Ohio St., Suite 600
Chicago, Ill. 60611-3201

Organizations

Agency for Health Care Policy and Research
18–12 Parklawn Bldg.
Rockville, Md. 20857

Computer-Based Patient Record Institute
919 North Michigan Ave.
Chicago, Ill. 60611-1683

National Library of Medicine
8600 Rockville Pike
Bethesda, Md. 20894

Conferences

The American Medical Informatics Association (AMIA) Spring Congress

The American Medical Informatics Association, Symposium on Computer Applications in Medical Care (SCAMC)

The Healthcare Information and Management Systems Society (HIMSS) Annual Conference

MEDINFO, sponsored by the International Medical Informatics Association

Journals

Communications of the Association for Computing Machinery

Computers and Biomedical Research

Health Affairs

Health Care Financing Review

Health Care Informatics

Health Policy and Law

Health Services Research

Hospitals and Health Networks

Inquiry

The Joint Commission Journal on Quality Improvement

Journal of the American Medical Association

Journal of the American Medical Informatics Association

MD Computing

The New England Journal of Medicine

Books

Blois, M. *Information and Medicine: The Nature of Medical Descriptions.* Berkeley and Los Angeles: University of California Press, 1984.

Blum, B. I., and Duncan, K. A. (eds.). *A History of Medical Informatics.* Reading, Mass.: Addison-Wesley, 1990.

Dick, R. S., and Steen, E. B. (eds.). *The Computer-Based Patient Record: An Essential Technology for Health Care.* Washington, D.C.: National Academy Press, 1991.

Katz, D., and Kahn, R. L. *The Social Psychology of Organizations.* (2nd ed.) New York: Wiley, 1978.

Shortliffe, E. H., Perreault, L. E., Wiederhold, G., and Fagan, L. M. (eds.). *Medical Informatics: Computer Applications in Health Care.* Reading, Mass.: Addison-Wesley, 1990.

Starr, P. *The Social Transformation of American Medicine.* New York: HarperCollins, 1984.

Weed, L. L. *Knowledge Coupling: New Premises and New Tools for Medical Care and Education.* New York: Springer-Verlag, 1991.

References

Anders, G. "Health-Care Firms Face Checkup for Merger Potential." *Wall Street Journal,* Oct. 12, 1993.

Andreopoulos, S. "Managed Health Care Competition Is Becoming a Scam." *San Jose Mercury News,* Feb. 17, 1993.

Austin, C. J. "Hospital Information Systems and the Development of a National Health Information System." In *Proceedings of the Fourteenth Hawaii International Conference on Systems Science.* N.p.: Western Periodicals Company, 1981.

Automated Medical Records: Leadership Needed to Expedite Standards Development. Washington, D.C.: U.S. Government Accounting Office, Apr. 1993.

Barnum, A. "Preventive Health Plan—Bay Firms Lead the Way." *San Francisco Chronicle,* Apr. 22, 1993.

Berwick, D. M., Godfrey, A. B., and Roessner, J. *Curing Health Care.* San Francisco: Jossey-Bass, 1990.

Blum, B. I., and Duncan, K. A. (eds.). *A History of Medical Informatics.* Reading, Mass.: ACM Press, Addison-Wesley, 1990.

Bria, W. "Look Doc, No Wires." *Healthcare Informatics,* May 1993, pp. 50–54.

Carlone, R. V. *Automated Medical Records: Leadership Needed to Expedite Standards Development.* Gaithersberg, Md.: U.S. General Accounting Office, Apr. 1993.

Clinton, J. J. "From the Agency for Health Care Policy and Research." *Journal of the American Medical Association,* 1993, *270*(12), 1405.

Computer-Based Patient Record Institute, Inc., Information Packet. Chicago: Computer-Based Patient Record Institute, 1993.

Cooper, H. "Health-Care Networks' Attempts to Cut Costs Are Trimming Patients' Options." *Wall Street Journal,* July 29, 1992.

A Coordinated Health Information System. Hearing before the Subcommittee on Science, Research and Technology of the Committee on Science and Technology, U.S. House of Representatives. Washington, D.C.: U.S. Government Printing Office, June 2–4, 1981.

Cotten, P. "Determining More Good Than Harm Is Not Easy." *Journal of the American Medical Association,* 1993, *270*(2), 153–158.

Demonstration and Evaluation of a Total Hospital Information System. Washington, D.C.: National Center for Health Services Research, July 1977.

Dick, R. S., and Steen, E. B. (eds.). *The Computer-Based Patient Record, An Essential Technology for Health Care.* Washington, D.C.: National Academy Press, 1991.

Ditto, W. L., and Pecora, L. M. "Mastering Chaos." *Scientific American,* Aug. 1993.

Duncan, K. A. "The Trend Toward a National Health Information System in the United States." In *Proceedings of Medinfo '80.* Amsterdam: North-Holland, 1980.

Duncan, K. A. *Planning and Research Agenda for a Coordinated Health Information System.* Testimony on a coordinated health information system before the Subcommittee on Science, Research and Technology of the Committee on Science and Technology, U.S. House of Representatives. Washington, D.C.: U.S. Government Printing Office, June 2–4, 1981.

Duncan, K. A. *Health Information Services: A Ten-Year Perspective.* San Jose, Calif.: Creative Strategies International, 1982.

Duncan, K. A. "Planning for Regional Health Information Services." In *Proceedings of Medinfo '83.* Amsterdam: North-Holland, 1983.

Duncan, K. A. "Medical Informatics: Clinical Decision Making and Beyond." In *Proceedings, American Association of Medical Systems and Informatics Congress 1988.* Washington, D.C.: American Medical Informatics Association, 1988.

Duncan, K. A. "A Perspective on Social Responsibility for the Computing Community." In *Education and Society, Proceedings of Information Processing 92.* Amsterdam: Elsevier Science, 1992.

Duncan, K. A., and others. *A Model Curriculum for Doctoral-Level Programs in Health Computing.* New York: Association for Computing Machinery, 1981.

Eddy, D. M., and Billings, J. "The Quality of Medical Evidence." *Health Affairs,* 1988, 7(1), 20.

Educating Medical Students. Assessing Change in Medical Education—The Road to Implementation (ACME-TRI) Report. Association of American Medical Colleges, 1992.

The Feasibility of Linking Research-Related Data Bases to Federal and Non-Federal Medical Administrative Data Bases. Rockville, Md.: Agency for Health Care Policy and Research, Public Health Service, Apr. 1991.

Foege, W. H. "Preventive Medicine and Public Health." *Journal of the American Medical Association,* 1992, *268*(3), 401–403.

Fowler, F. J., Jr. *Health Survey Research Methods.* Washington, D.C.: National Center for Health Services Research, Sept. 1989.

Franks, P., Nutting, P. A., and Clancy, C. M. "Health Care Reform, Primary Care, and the Need for Research." *Journal of the American Medical Association,* 1993, *270*(12), 1449–1453.

Ginsberg, E. "Physician Supply Policies and Health Reform." *Journal of the American Medical Association,* 1992, *268*(21), 3115–3118.

Giovannucci, E., and others. "A Prospective Cohort Study of

Vasectomy and Prostate Cancer in US Men." *Journal of the American Medical Association,* 1993a, *269*(7), 873–877.

Giovannucci, E., and others. "A Retrospective Cohort Study of Vasectomy and Prostate Cancer in US Men." *Journal of the American Medical Association,* 1993b, *269*(7), 878–882.

Grady, M. L., and Schwartz, H. A. *Medical Effectiveness Research Data Methods.* Rockville, Md.: Agency for Health Care Policy and Research, Public Health Service, July 1992.

Grimes, D. A. "Technology Follies: The Uncritical Acceptance of Medical Innovation." *Journal of the American Medical Association,* 1993, *269*(23), 3030–3033.

"Health Net Execs May Reap Millions on Merger." *San Francisco Chronicle,* Sept. 2, 1993.

"HMOs Expecting Business to Boom." *San Francisco Chronicle,* May 13, 1993.

"Improving Health Professionals' Access to Information." In *National Library of Medicine Long-Range Plan.* Bethesda, Md.: National Institutes of Health, Aug. 1989.

Jarvinen, P. "Impacts of Electronic Markets on Work." In *Education and Society, Proceedings of Information Processing 92.* Amsterdam: Elsevier Science, 1992.

Jones, D. "Hospital Company Chief to Challenge Clinton." *USA Today,* Oct. 12, 1993.

Kaple, J. M. "Health Information Systems for the 1980's." In *Proceedings of the Fourteenth Hawaii International Conference on Systems Science.* N.p.: Western Periodicals Company, 1981.

Klainer, L. M. "The VA's Emerging National Health Information System." In *Proceedings of the Fourteenth Hawaii International Conference on Systems Science.* N.p.: Western Periodicals Company, 1981.

Laffel, G., and Berwick, D. M. "Quality in Health Care." *Journal of the American Medical Association,* 1992, *268*(3), 407–409.

McKenney, J. L. *Waves of Change: Business Evolution Through Information Technology.* Cambridge, Mass.: Harvard University Press, 1994.

National Cholesterol Education Program. "Summary of the Second Report of the NCEP Expert Panel on Detection, Evaluation, and Treatment of High Blood Cholesterol in Adults." *Journal of the American Medical Association,* 1993, *269*(23), 3015–3022.

Owens, D. K., and Nease, R. F., Jr. "Development of Outcome-Based Practice Guidelines: A Method for Structuring Problems and Synthesizing Evidence." *Journal on Quality Improvement,* 1993, *19*(7), 248–263.

Parasuraman, S., and others. "Automation-Related Complacency: A Source of Vulnerability in Contemporary Organizations." In *Education and Society, Proceedings of Information Processing 92.* Amsterdam: Elsevier Science, 1992.

Petit, C. "Genentech Beats Cheaper Rival in Battle of Heart Attack Drugs." *San Francisco Chronicle,* May 1, 1993.

Priester, R. "A Values Framework for Health System Reform." *Health Affairs,* 1992, *11*(1), 84–107.

Raskin, I. E., and Maklan, C. W. *Medical Treatment Effectiveness Research.* Rockville, Md.: Agency for Health Care Policy and Research, Public Health Service, 1991.

Robitaille, S. "Auditors Suspend ProCare." *San Jose Mercury News,* Mar. 25, 1993.

Salive, M. E., Mayfield, J. A., and Weissman, N. W. "Patient Outcomes Research Teams and the Agency for Health Care Policy and Research." *Health Services Research,* 1990, *25*(5), 697–708.

Schiller, Z. "Humana Wheels Itself to Surgery." *Business Week,* Jan. 25, 1993.

Schoenbaum, S. C. "Toward Fewer Procedures and Better Outcomes." *Journal of the American Medical Association,* 1993, *2269*(6), 794–796.

Sechrest, L., Perrin, E., and Bunker, J. *Research Methodology: Strengthening Causal Interpretations of Nonexperimental Data.* Rockville, Md.: Agency for Health Care Policy and Research, Public Health Service, May 1990.

Shannon, R. H. "The Barrier at the Top." In *Proceedings of the*

Fourteenth Hawaii International Conference on Systems Science. N.p.: Western Periodicals Company, 1981.

Shannon, R. H. "Hierarchies, the Health Field, and Curricula." In J. C. Pages, A. H. Levy, F. Gremy, and J. Anderson (eds.), *Meeting the Challenge: Informatics and Medical Education.* Amsterdam: North-Holland, 1983.

Siu, A. L., and others. "Choosing Quality of Care Measures Based on the Expected Impact of Improved Care on Health." *Health Services Research,* 1992, *27*(5), 610–650.

Skolnick, A. A. "Joint Commission Will Collect, Publicize Outcomes." *Journal of the American Medical Association,* 1993, *270*(2), 165–171.

Starr, P. *The Social Transformation of American Medicine.* New York: Basic Books, 1982.

Stead, W. W., and others. "The IAIMS at Duke University Medical Center: Transition from Model Testing to Implementation." *M.D. Computing,* 1993, *10*(4), 225–230.

Steinmetz, G. "New York Life Reaches an Agreement to Expand Its Managed-Care Business." *Wall Street Journal,* Sept. 22, 1993.

"A Vision of the Future." In *Long Range Plan: Medical Informatics.* Bethesda, Md.: National Library of Medicine, 1986.

Wagner, I. "Vulnerability of Computer Systems: Establishing Organizational Accountability." In *Education and Society, Proceedings of Information Processing 92.* Amsterdam: Elsevier Science, 1992.

Weed, L. L. "Medical Records That Guide and Teach." *M.D. Computing,* 1993, *10*(2), 110–114. (Originally published in 1968.)

Wennberg, J. E. "Improving the Medical Decision-Making Process." *Health Affairs,* 1988, 7(1), 99–106.

Wennberg, J. E., Freeman, F. L., and Culp, W. J. "Are Hospital Services Rationed in New Haven or Over-Utilized in Boston?" *Lancet,* May 23, 1987, pp. 1185–1188.

Williams, B. T., Imrey, H., and Williams, R. G. "The Lifespan Personal Health Record." *Medical Decision Making,* 1991, *11*(suppl.), S74–S76.

Young, E.W.D. *Alpha and Omega*. Reading, Mass.: Addison-Wesley, 1989.

Zaldivar, R. A. "The Cost of Caring." *San Jose Mercury News,* July 11, 1993.

Zengerle, P. "Virtual Reality Gets Serious." *San Francisco Examiner,* Aug. 22, 1993.

Index

A

Access to care: evolution of, 45–47, 57; issue of, 86–87

Accessibility of information: concept of, 98; in information framework, 134; logjam in, 104–105; in patient record, 229

Accountability, and administrative waste, 68–69

Accreditation, role of, 90

Administrative waste, issue of, 68–69

Administrators, in networks, 259–260

Agency for Health Care Policy and Research (AHCPR): address of, 316; and clinical guidelines, 298; Medical Treatment Effectiveness Program of, 268–269; Patient Outcomes Research Teams of, 270; and primary care, 300

Aggregation: configurations for, 179–188; in information framework, 148, 150–155, 156–157, 158; by information service centers, 194; in networks, 207, 212, 218; of patient records, 102–104, 122, 139–140

American Airlines, 163, 202

American Healthcare Information Management Association, 315

American Hospital Supply, 164

American Medical Association: and national policy, 10, 36, 45, 53; as trade association, 53, 90, 228

American Medical Informatics Association, 315, 316

American National Standards Institute, 269

American Society for Testing and Materials, 269

American Specialists Association, 157–158

Anders, G., 53

Andreopoulos, S., 59

Association for Computing Machinery, Education Board of, 273

Association for Health Services Research, 315

327